101

Frequently Asked Questions about "Health & Fitness" and "Nutrition & Weight Control"

Cedric X. Bryant, Ph.D, FACSM
James A. Peterson, Ph.D, FACSM
Barry A. Franklin, Ph.D, FACSM

Foreword by H. Thomas Bryant
President and CEO
StairMaster Sports/Medical Products, Inc.

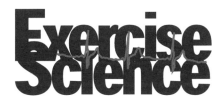

ISBN: 1-57167-452-7
Library of Congress Card Catalog Number: 99-62748

Cover Design: Jennifer Bokelmann, Jennie Scott
Interior Design: Michelle Summers, Jim Wilkerson
Cover Photos: StairMaster Sports Medical Products Inc. (upper left, lower
                right); Comstock, Inc. (lower left, upper right)

Exercise Science is a division of: Sagamore Publishing, Inc.
                                        P.O. Box 647
                                        Champaign, IL 61824-0647
                                        Web Site: http//www.sagamorepub.com

Dedication

To those members of the exercise science and medical communities whose efforts and professionalism over the years have enabled individuals to better understand both the countless benefits of exercise and how those benefits can be achieved through a combination of sound exercise and healthy eating habits. We commend those who have made a resolute commitment to a wellness-oriented lifestyle. Hopefully this book will help facilitate their task in this regard.

Contents

Foreword

Since our inception in 1983, StairMaster® Sports/Medical Products, Inc., has been firmly committed to providing the best products and service to those organizations and individuals who want innovative, well-designed exercise equipment of the highest quality. As an integral part of that commitment, StairMaster has undertaken a number of steps to ensure that its products are extraordinarily safe, and to inform its customers of the substantial benefits of sound exercise.

In 1989, for example, StairMaster established an in-house Department of Sports Medicine—the only such department in the health-fitness industry. Currently, this department is staffed by trained exercise and sports-medicine scientists, including a fellow of the prestigious American College of Sports Medicine (ACSM) and the co-editor of ACSM's *Guidelines for Exercise Testing and Prescription, 5th Edition*. Consistent with its commitment to develop medically sound products, the company's in-house research facilities include a state-of-the-art physiological and biomechanical testing laboratory for conducting pilot studies, evaluating equipment design, and determining the accuracy and reliability of the performance and physiological feedback provided by its products.

Among the other actions taken by StairMaster to reinforce its "sports/medical emphasis" have been to institute and support an extensive program of independently conducted research studies at such renowned institutions as Harvard University, Stanford University, the U.S. Military Academy, the Cleveland Clinic, and the U.S. Olympic Training Center. To date, more than 150 studies have been conducted. We have developed and distributed wellness-based educational materials that have been made available to anyone requesting them–particularly those in the health and fitness industry. In addition, we continue to sponsor educational symposia, colloquia, and clinics.

It is our belief that *101 Frequently Asked Questions about "Health & Fitness" and "Nutrition & Weight Control"* is yet another example of the consistent effort by StairMaster to provide useful resources to individuals interested in health and fitness. We hope that this book helps to reinforce the fact that when you think of health and fitness, you think of StairMaster. Enjoy.

H. Thomas Bryant
President and CEO
StairMaster Sports/Medical Products, Inc.

About the Authors

Cedric X. Bryant, Ph.D., FACSM, is the senior vice president of research and development/sports medicine at StairMaster Sports/Medical Products, Inc., Kirkland, Washington. Barry A. Franklin, Ph.D., FACSM, is director of the Cardiac Rehabilitation and Exercise Laboratories, William Beaumont Hospital, and Professor of Physiology, Wayne State University, School of Medicine, Detroit, Michigan. James A. Peterson, Ph.D., FACSM, is a sports medicine specialist residing in Monterey, California. All three authors are fellows and active members of the American College of Sports Medicine (ACSM) and internationally known authors and speakers on topics relating to fitness and nutrition. Dr. Franklin is currently the president of ACSM.

Part 1:
Health and Fitness

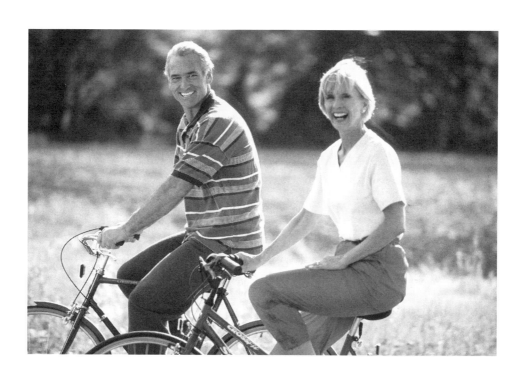

FAQ #1

Question: Does any proof exist that exercise can help a person live longer?

Answer: Absolutely. In fact, the largest study measuring fitness ever conducted found that regular exercise will indeed help a person live longer. Led by Dr. Steven Blair of the Institute of Aerobics Research in Dallas, the eight-year study evaluated the fitness and mortality levels of 13,344 men and women. Researchers involved with the study found that exercise reduces the death rate from all causes, particularly cancer and heart disease. Physical fitness was measured by each subject's performance on a standardized treadmill test—a test which is designed to accurately assess aerobic fitness (the most commonly accepted indicator of cardiorespiratory fitness). Based on the test results, the subjects were then grouped by gender into five categories ranging from least to most fit.

The results of the study, which were published in the *Journal of the American Medical Association*, showed that the higher the fitness level the lower the death rate, after the data were adjusted for age differences between the subjects. Compared with the most-fit subjects, individuals in the least-fit category had death rates 3.4 and 4.6 times higher for men and women respectively. The differences in mortality rates held relatively constant even after adjustments for coronary risk factors, such as smoking and cholesterol level, were considered. For both men and women, the largest drop from one fitness category to another was from the least-fit to the next most-fit group. Expressed as deaths per 10,000 person-years, the age-adjusted death rates for men and women in the sedentary category fell from 64 and 39.5 to 25.5 and 20.5 respectively in the next most-fit group, a decline of more than 60 percent for men and 48 percent for women.

The implication of Blair's findings are extraordinarily significant, particularly for a sedentary individual. On a major scale, this study documents the fact that a modest amount of exercise can and does go a long way. The equivalent of brisk walking 30 minutes a day is all that is required to move from the most sedentary category to the next most fit category.

FAQ #2

Question: Should I be concerned with the fact that I experience headaches when I exercise?

Answer: The majority of headaches associated with exercise are benign. The most common example of this type of headache is the so-called "exertion headache." Researchers suggest (but are not certain) that exertion headaches are vascular in origin—caused by the abrupt dilation or constriction of blood vessels. More often than not, these headaches occur just after exercise and may be quite painful. Fortunately, with rest, the pain goes away.

Another type of headache that is associated with exercise is potentially much more serious. If you are over the age of 50, have headaches that begin during exercise and go away with rest, *and* you have specific risk factors for heart disease (e.g., high blood pressure, diabetes, smoking, family history of heart disease, etc.), your headaches may be a sign of heart disease. The key point to remember is that individuals with cardiac headaches may not experience other outward signs of heart disease. As such, if you suffer from the aforementioned risk factors for heart disease and you are experiencing headaches that are brought on by exercise, you should consult your physician.

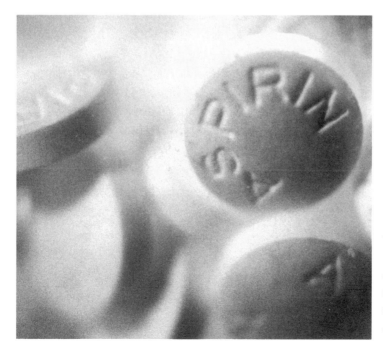

The majority of headaches associated with exercise are benign.

FAQ #3

Question: What is exercise- induced amenorrhea and is it dangerous?

Answer: Women who engage in intense exercise training may stop having their periods altogether—a condition known as amenorrhea. While the absence of the menstrual period may appear to present less of a problem to a woman than having to contend with the associated signs and symptoms, it is very important to determine why the menstrual period has ceased. Amenorrhea is a relatively pervasive condition. Approximately two to five percent of the general female populations and up to 43 percent of athletic women do not have menstrual periods. Amenorrhea, however, is not exclusive to athletes; other factors have also been found to cause amenorrhea, including pregnancy, very early menopause, anorexia nervosa, and certain types of tumors.

The cause of exercise-induced amenorrhea is still not fully understood, but contributing factors include excessive weight loss/thinness, age, a previous history of menstrual abnormalities, and diet—not to mention the intensity, duration, and frequency of exercise. While amenorrhea can occur in any sport, the incidence of amenorrhea is particularly high in participants in gymnastics, distance running, ballet, and figure skating.

Why all the concern about amenorrhea? Since the 1980's, research has been conducted that has linked amenorrhea to low estrogen levels. Because estrogen is essential for developing and maintaining normal bone health, low levels of estrogen can reflect serious deficits. The process by which your basic skeleton is formed (i.e., via the deposit of calcium into the bone cells) is generally completed by age 35. Theoretically, therefore, if you don't deposit adequate levels of calcium in your bones as a young woman, you may develop osteoporosis (i.e., decreased bone mass and increased susceptibility to fractures) at an earlier age than normal and, worse yet, your case may be more severe. Regrettably, osteoporosis affects over 30 million Americans annually.

FAQ #4

Question: What effect, if any, does smoking have on my running performance?

Answer: Research has established that smoking impairs an individual's ability to perform vigorous exercise because of an increased level of carbon monoxide in the blood, a reduced level of lung function, and a decreased level of maximal oxygen uptake. Carbon monoxide primarily affects exercise performance through its strong (i.e., 200 times stronger than that of oxygen) capacity to bind to hemoglobin in the blood, thereby reducing the blood's capacity to transport oxygen. This factor decreases the delivery of oxygen to the muscles during vigorous exercise, making all effort seem more difficult than normal. At rest, and to a lesser extent during exercise, nicotine from cigarette smoke increases heart rate, blood pressure, and the oxygen demands of the heart. During exercise, nicotine also increases the blood levels of lactic acid—a substance that can cause individuals to feel fatigued when it rises to relatively high levels. In studies conducted on animals, nicotine has been shown to impair high endurance exercise capacity (essential for long duration running or swimming). The resistance to airflow following smoking is increased in the passageways of the lungs, making it more difficult to deliver air and oxygen to the lungs during strenuous exercise. In some individuals, cigarette smoke can trigger asthma-like symptoms, making it virtually impossible to exercise until the symptoms disappear.

In general, most health and fitness experts believe that when compared with nonsmokers, smokers are less fit to start with because of their smoking habit, and then lose more fitness and lung function with the passage of time. Scientists who have compared the fitness of smokers and non-smokers, for example, report that smokers come out on the short end. In a study of 1,000 relatively young Air Force recruits, Dr. Kenneth Cooper found that the ability to run as far as possible in 12 minutes was inversely related to the number of cigarettes smoked, with those smoking more than 30 cigarettes a day exhibiting the poorest run performance.

FAQ #5

Question: My doctor tells me I have chondromalacia. What should I do about it?

Answer: Chondromalacia, commonly referred to as runner's or jumper's knee, is a fairly prevalent condition in which repeated stress on the knee causes inflammation and an eventual softening of the cartilage under the kneecap (patella). In turn, this condition has an adverse effect on the smooth gliding of the kneecap that normally occurs over the end of the femur. Eventually, a roughness, pain, or swelling of the knee may develop. Symptoms can occur underneath or on both sides of the kneecap. Treating chondromalacia is a fairly straightforward undertaking. If your knee is painful and swollen, you should incorporate an appropriate amount of rest into your regimen. You should also apply ice to your knee at least twice a day for approximately 15 minutes each time. Most physicians also recommend taking anti-inflammatory drugs (e.g., aspirin, ibuprofen, etc.). With regard to continuing to exercise, you should let pain be your guide. If the pain in your kneecap is aggravated by exercising, you should either decrease the amount or the level of intensity of your exercise activity or switch to a non-weight bearing activity (e.g., swimming). If the pain then persists, you should see your physician for further advice.

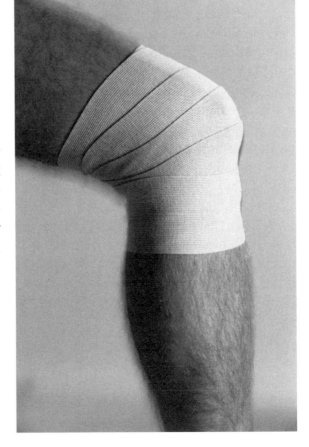

If the pain in your kneecap is aggravated by exercising, you should either decrease the amount or the level of intensity of your exercise activity or switch to a non-weight bearing activity (e.g., swimming).

FAQ #6

Question: What is athlete's foot and how can it be prevented?

Answer: Athlete's foot is a fungal infection spread either from person-to-person or by direct contact with a contaminated surface (e.g., shower mat, locker room carpet, towel, etc.). Among the more effective preventive measures for athlete's foot are the following:

- Keep the feet as dry as possible.
- Wear "breathable" socks (i.e., cotton or wool) and change them frequently (e.g., one to three times per day).
- Wear shower sandals (i.e., don't go barefoot) in the locker room or shower.
- Avoid wearing restrictive footwear or plastic insoles.
- Alternate wearing pairs of sneakers, if possible.
- Use antifungal sprays, powders, or lotions.

FAQ #7

Question: Does regular participation in aerobic exercise lower an individual's risk of developing cancer?

Answer: While it has not been shown that a given level of physical activity per se can reduce overall cancer risk, research suggests that exercise often modifies some of the risk factors associated with certain kinds of cancer. Obesity, for example, has been linked to cancer of the breast and the female reproductive system. In turn, regular exercise has been shown to help promote weight loss. Several studies have also found that men who worked at sedentary jobs for most of their lives had a greater incidence of colon cancer than those in more active jobs. A longitudinal study of Harvard alumni found that highly active or even moderately active individuals had a substantially lower risk of developing both colon and lung cancer than alumni who were less active or sedentary. On the other hand, exercise will not offset the effects of a high-fat diet or cigarette smoking. Still, it can contribute, even indirectly, to a reduced risk of cancer. As such, exercising regularly is recommended by the American Cancer Society as an integral part of its cancer prevention program.

FAQ #8

Question: Can you offer some basic guidelines for avoiding overuse injuries associated with running?

Answer: Generally speaking, the vast majority of overuse injuries associated with running can be avoided by utilizing common sense and not exposing your body to sudden, high levels of orthopedic stress. Among some of the more basic guidelines for sidestepping running-related overuse injuries are the following:

Stretch before and after exercising. Proper stretching can mean the difference between agony and enjoyment. Such stretching can have several benefits, including increasing the range of motion of your musculature, reducing your chances of being injured, and improving your level of performance. As a general rule, always precede your stretching exercises with at least three to five minutes of low-intensity aerobic activity.

- Stretch before and after exercising. Proper stretching can mean the difference between agony and enjoyment. According to a new ACSM position stand, stretching can have several benefits, including increasing the range of motion of your musculature, reducing your chances of being injured, and improving your level of performance. As a general rule, always precede your stretching exercises with at least three to five minutes of low-intensity aerobic activity.

- Increase your mileage sensibly. Avoid doing too much exercise too soon. A general guideline is to limit any increase in your weekly distance to ten percent or less of your previous week's total mileage. Contrary to the opinion of some overzealous enthusiasts, exercise is not a contest. The quality of exercise is often more important than the quantity of physical activity.

- Incorporate a relatively "easy" week into your exercise regimen every so often. Keep in mind that you don't have to increase your mileage every week to continue to benefit from your efforts.

- Don't subject your body to consecutive days of very intense exercise. Always follow a relatively "hard" day of exercising with an easier day. If you run considerably further than usual on a particular day, either take the next day off or decrease the duration and intensity of your next workout.

- Treat all injuries immediately and properly. As a general guideline, the acronym "RICE" should serve as the basis of treatment for most minor injuries (e.g., pulled or strained muscles, shin splints, etc.)— rest, ice, compression, and elevation.

- Don't ignore sudden, acute pain. See a physician—preferably a sports medicine specialist—if your acute pain does not respond to self-treatment within a reasonable period of time. The point to remember is that you must listen to your body. Keep in mind that pain is your body's early warning signal that something is wrong. Pain is your body's way of telling you that if you persist in what you're doing, you will either injure yourself or will compound a relatively minor injury which has already occurred.

- Limit your total weekly mileage to an appropriate (i.e., reasonable) level. If you exercise too much, you substantially increase your chances of suffering an overuse injury.

- Replace your shoes periodically. Proper footwear can have a significant impact on minimizing your likelihood of injury. You should record your mileage daily and replace your shoes once the cumulative total on a particular pair exceeds 500 miles.

- Don't let pain change your natural pattern of movement while exercising. If you alter your normal foot plant while running in an effort to adjust for pain or discomfort, you may place excessive stress on your joints and the adjacent tendons, ligaments, and musculature. You should refrain from exercising until the pain subsides and no longer interferes with your natural walking or running mechanics.

- Vary your modality of training. Give the joints and muscles of your body an occasional break from the "same old grind." Engage in other forms of exercise (e.g., cycling, swimming, stair climbing, rowing, etc.) in addition to running.

FAQ #9

Question: What is runner's knee and how is it treated?

Answer: The medical term for runner's knee is patellofemoral syndrome. This injury is the most common in runners and accounts for up to 30 percent of all running injuries. The pain is thought to emanate from nerve fibers in the subchondral bone of the patella or from a synovitis (i.e., inflammation of a synovial membrane). It is typically characterized by a dull pain located behind the kneecap. It also tends to have a gradual onset and is usually exacerbated by ascending or descending stairs or by downhill running. Individuals suffering from patellofemoral syndrome often experience stiffness when straightening the knee after sitting for extended periods of time. Rest and the application of ice are typically the first treatment options for this overuse injury. An additional goal of therapy for this condition also includes correcting misalignment of the patella by developing the vastus medialis oblique muscle of the quadriceps. This objective can be accomplished by performing a series of exercises, such as wall slides, end-range leg extensions, and end-range leg presses.

· ·

FAQ #10

Question: Can aerobic exercise have a positive effect in preventing or eliminating headache pain?

Answer: Research indicates that headache sufferers who improve their baseline levels of physical fitness and muscle tone, as a general rule, have fewer and less severe bouts of pain. This relationship appears to apply to almost all of the various types of headaches. Sound aerobic exercise causes the brain to secrete more endorphins and enkephalins—the body's own opiate-like, pain-dampening chemicals. As the number of headache-slaying chemicals produced by the body increases, the body's threshold for pain incurs a similar increase. It is important to note, however, that aerobic exercise tends to help tension headache sufferers more than those experiencing migraines, although low-impact, low-intensity exercise at the first sign of a migraine may be beneficial.

FAQ #11

Question: My doctor recommends that I fill out a health-risk appraisal (HRA) form and have him evaluate my health status before I begin an aerobic exercise program. What is an HRA and do you think I need one?

Answer: For most individuals, aerobic exercise is a very safe endeavor. For a few people, however, vigorous exercise can involve a substantial degree of risk. These primarily include persons with documented or occult heart disease who are habitually sedentary. Accordingly, it is advisable that *all* adults undergo some type of pre-activity HRA before initiating an aerobic exercise program and, on a periodic basis thereafter, to identify any subsequent changes in the individual's health status, signified by abnormal signs or symptoms. A pre-activity HRA is important for a number of reasons, including:

- to identify and exclude individuals with medical contraindications to exercise.

- to assure the safety of exercise testing and training programs.

- to determine the appropriate exercise test or exercise program for an individual.

- to identify individuals with clinically significant diseases who should be referred to a medically supervised exercise program.

- to identify individuals with either disease symptoms or risk factors for disease who should receive further medical evaluation before initiating an exercise program.

- to identify individuals who have special needs that might preclude them from safely participating in physical activity.

- to provide information that might serve as the basis for advice given to an individual regarding the relationship between good health and that person's behavior as it relates to physical activity and the risk of developing heart disease, orthopedic problems, metabolic conditions, or other diseases.

- to obtain information to motivate an individual toward meaningful life-style changes.

FAQ #12

Question: What is overtraining? Are there any easy-to-recognize signs or symptoms of overtraining?

Answer: Overtraining is a term that is used to express a situation when an imbalance occurs between training and recovery. The symptoms of overtraining can vary from one individual to another. Overtraining, however, frequently involves one or more of the following common signs or symptoms:

- impaired physical performance

- reduced enthusiasm and desire for training

- increased resting heart rate (i.e., your heart rate taken first thing in the morning before getting out of bed)

- increased resting blood pressure

- chronic muscle or joint soreness

- increased incidence of musculoskeletal injuries

- increased incidence of colds and infections

- impaired recovery from exercise (e.g., heart rate remains elevated well after the completion of a bout of exercise)

- increased perceived exertion during your normal workouts

- reduced appetite

- dramatic weight loss

- disturbed sleep patterns

- increased depression, irritability, or anxiety

FAQ #13

Question: I recently tore my knee up in a skiing accident. Is there anything I can do while I am rehabbing my knee to maintain my level of aerobic fitness?

Answer: Fortunately, despite the fact that most people tend to view aerobic training as merely a lower extremity form of exercise, you can exercise aerobically by using your upper body. Aerobically training your upper body, however, is a far more challenging task than aerobically training your lower body (basically because of the disproportionately less muscle mass you have in your arms compared to your legs). The primary keys to achieving a satisfactory training effect from your upper body aerobic exercise efforts are to exercise at an appropriate training heart rate (i.e., the prescribed exercise heart rate for leg training should be reduced by approximately 10 bpm for arm training), to exercise at a suitable work rate (i.e., a work rate approximately 50 percent of that used for leg training is generally appropriate for arm training), and to select an exercise modality that will enable you to achieve your goals (e.g., arm crank ergometer, Versaclimber, StairMaster Crossrobics® Kayak™, etc.).

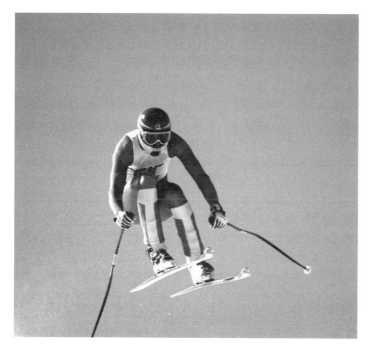

Aerobically training your upper body, however, is a far more challenging task than aerobically training your lower body.

FAQ #14

Question: Who should have an exercise stress test and how safe is such a test?

Answer: The current guidelines of American Heart Association indicate that if you are under age 40 (male and female) and undergo a normal physical examination, which indicates no symptoms of cardiovascular disease, no major coronary risk factors, no physical findings (including murmurs and hypertension), you are likely free of disease and do not require an exercise stress test before undertaking a vigorous exercise regimen. If you are 40 years of age or older, have had an abnormal physical examination (murmurs, etc.) or possess two or more major coronary risk factors, you should have an exercise stress test before embarking on a vigorous exercise program (refer to Table 2 for a listing of the primary coronary risk factors).

In guidelines recently revised by the American College of Sports Medicine (ACSM), an exercise stress test is not recommended prior to initiation of an exercise program if you are an asymptomatic male 40 years or younger, or female 50 years or younger. If you are an older asymptomatic adult (males 40 plus, females 50 plus), you may initiate a moderate exercise regimen (intensity 40-60 percent $\dot{V}O_2$ max) without an exercise stress test. An exercise stress test is recommended for all older adults planning a vigorous exercise program (intensity greater than 60 percent $\dot{V}O_2$ max).

The ACSM uses the same criteria of two or more major coronary risk factors as the basis for recommending an exercise stress test prior to an individual's beginning an exercise program. Gradual moderate exercise is, however, permitted without an exercise stress test for individuals without coronary artery disease (CAD) symptoms, but with two or more CAD risk factors. Individuals with two or more major coronary risk factors, but without symptoms, should undergo an exercise stress test before vigorous exercise. Moreover, individuals of any age with documented cardiopulmonary or metabolic disease (or symptoms suggestive of disease–e.g., chest pain, light headedness, palpitations) should undergo a physical examination and an exercise stress test before embarking on a vigorous exercise program.

Like most medical procedures, an exercise stress test is not without some risk. The risk can be minimized by proper screening and by having the test administered by properly trained personnel. Although unexpected events (e.g., cardiovascular complications) are well publicized, they are extremely rare (approximately 9 per 10,000 symptom-limited exercise stress tests). The risk of a fatality while engaging in an exercise stress tests in a clinic is much lower (less than 1 in 10,000).

Table 1. Coronary Artery Disease Risk Factors*

Positive Risk Factors	Defining Criteria
1. Age	Men >45 years; women >55 or premature menopause without estrogen replacement therapy
2. Family history	Myocardial infraction or sudden death before 55 years of age in father or other male first-degree relative, or before 65 years of age in mother or other female first-degree relative
3. Current cigarette smoking	
4. Hypertension	Blood pressure >140/90 mm Hg, confirmed by measurements on at least 2 separate occasions, or on antihypertensive medication
5. Hypercholesterolemia	Total serum cholesterol >200 mg/dL (5.2 mmol/L) (if lipoprotein profile is unavailable) or HDL <35 mg/dL (0.9 mmol/L)
6. Diabetes mellitus	Persons with insulin dependent diabetes mellitus (IDDM) who are >30 years of age, or have had IDDM for >15 years, and persons with non-insulin dependent diabetes mellitus (NIDDM) who are >35 years of age should be classified as patients with disease
7. Sedentary life-style /physical inactivity	Persons comprising the least active 25 percent of the population, as defined by the combination of sedentary jobs involving sitting for a large part of the day and no regular exercise or active recreational pursuits

* Adapted in part from the *Journal of the American Medical Association 269*:3015-3023, 1993.

FAQ #15

Question: Do the benefits of aerobic dancing outweigh the potential risks associated with it?

Answer: In most cases, they do—particularly when the participant takes a sensible approach to exercising, such as adhering to the following general guidelines:

- Don't try to do too much too soon.

- Build up gradually in both intensity and duration.

- Make sure that the body is up for the stresses imposed by the aerobic dancing (e.g., strengthen the muscles supporting the ligaments involved in the exercise).

- Warm up and stretch before exercising.

- Learn and practice biomechanically correct techniques and movements for the exercise.

While, by definition, exercise involves stress to your body and without such stress your body would not make the physiological adaptations that enable you to improve your fitness level, it is neither sensible nor productive to push your body beyond the limits it can reasonably sustain. Aerobic dancing has been shown to produce a demonstrable training effect when participants adhere to appropriate levels of intensity, frequency, and duration. The risk of injury associated with aerobic dance can never be entirely eliminated, but most of the potential problems may be avoided simply by using "common sense" and listening to your body's important warning signals (pain, discomfort, excessive fatigue, etc.).

-

FAQ #16

Question: What steps can an individual take to avoid heat injury when exercising in a relatively hot environment?

Answer: A potential health hazard of exercising in warm weather exercise is heat injury. A key point to remember is that anyone who exercises in a hot environment is susceptible to heat injury. In the excessively warm and often humid conditions that frequently occur in the summer and early fall, heat stress can be a real threat for individuals who engage in aerobic-type exercise activities—either outdoors or indoors in facilities without air conditioning.

Individuals exercising in a warm, humid environment should adhere to five relatively basic guidelines to avoid heat injury. First, make sure that they are adequately hydrated. This can be accomplished by consuming copious amounts of fluid (just short of feeling fully bloated) thirty minutes before exercise, drinking at least six ounces of fluid after approximately every 20 minutes of exercise, and drinking beyond thirst cessation during the recovery period. Water is generally considered the best hydration fluid unless the duration of the exercise bout exceeds 90 minutes. If an individual exercises for longer than an hour and a half, a diluted commercial beverage may be the most appropriate fluid to consume.

Second, an individual should become acclimatized to the environment. Acclimatization, the body's gradual adaptation to changes in environment (it usually takes 10-14 days of heat exposure combined with exercise), can greatly reduce an individual's risk for heat injury. Following acclimatization, individuals will sweat sooner, produce more sweat, and lose less electrolytes in their sweat. The net effects of acclimatization are a lower body core temperature, a decreased heart rate response to exercise, and a diminished potential for dehydration and electrolyte depletion. Third, individuals should lower the intensity level of their exercise bout (especially during the acclimatization period) because this step will decrease the heat load and reduce the strain on their thermoregulatory mechanisms.

Fourth, individuals should never wear clothing that is impermeable to water (e.g., rubberized sweat suits), since such clothing prevents the evaporation of sweat from the skin and thereby increase the risk of heat injury. Fifth, every individual should respect the existing environmental conditions since temperature and relative humidity can greatly influence both the degree of heat stress and the body's ability to effectively respond to the heat stress. As a general rule of thumb, an individual should consider curtailing exercise when the ambient temperature is above 90 degrees Fahrenheit and, concurrently, the relative humidity is above 60 percent. In summation, warm weather exercisers should adhere to the following motto: "drink up, slow down, and have fun exercising."

FAQ #17

Question: What constitutes an appropriate aerobic exercise prescription for a pregnant woman?

Answer: The ACOG has established guidelines (refer to Table 2) for aerobic exercise during pregnancy and the postpartum period. These advisory instructions are intended to be suitable for all pregnant women regardless of their basic level of physical fitness. Many leading authorities, however, believe that the ACOG guidelines are too conservative and that a more appropriate exercise prescription for a pregnant woman would be one that is more individualized. These experts feel that decisions related to the type, intensity, duration, and frequency of exercise should be made according to a women's current fitness level, the stage of her pregnancy, and her personal interests.

It appears that some exercise activities are more suitable than others for a pregnant woman who is just beginning an exercise program. The most suitable aerobic exercises for the newly exercising pregnant woman are low-impact activities such as walking, swimming, cycling, and independent-action, machine-based stair climbing. Women accustomed to running prior to pregnancy can safely continue to do so provided they "listen to their bodies." All factors considered, the most appropriate form of aerobic exercise for a pregnant woman is the one that she most enjoys and can safely perform.

The fundamental purpose of exercise during pregnancy is to maintain or improve fitness. Thus, the intensity, frequency, and duration at which exercise is prescribed for a pregnant woman should be adjusted downward. An appropriate level of exercise intensity for a pregnant woman is 50 percent of maximal oxygen uptake, or resting heart rate plus 50-60 percent of the difference between resting and maximal heart rate. If, however, a pregnant woman is unable to comfortably carry on a conversation while exercising (a.k.a. the "talk test"), she should reduce her exercise work rate. The "talk test" tends to err on the side of conservatism and can be very helpful in ensuring that the intensity of an exercise bout is not excessive for a particular individual at a particular moment in time. As far as exercise frequency and duration are concerned, it is suggested that a healthy pregnant woman exercise at least three times per week (non-consecutive days) for 20-30 minutes per session. Some examples (e.g., Joan Benoit Samuelson) exist of women who are able to engage in more intense, more frequent, and longer bouts of exercise.

It is the opinion of many experts that an individualized exercise prescription is safer and more effective for the vast majority of pregnant women. Over the course of their pregnancies, most women appear to spontaneously adjust the intensity, duration, and/or frequency of their workouts to appropriate levels (e.g., most women tend to naturally exercise at lower intensities and for shorter durations during the latter stages of pregnancy). A good indicator of an appropriate exercise prescription is that a pregnant woman should be fully recovered within 15-20 minutes after the workout.

Table 2. American College of Obstetricians and Gynecologists (ACOG) Recommendations for Exercise in Pregnancy and Postpartum*

1.	During pregnancy, women can continue to exercise and derive health benefits even from mild-to-moderate exercise routines. Regular exercise (at least three times per week) is preferable to intermittent activity.
2.	Women should avoid exercise in the supine position after the first trimester. This position is associated with decreased cardiac output in most pregnant women; because the remaining cardiac output will be preferentially distributed away from splanchnic beds (including the uterus) during vigorous exercise, such regimens are best avoided during pregnancy. Prolonged periods of motionless standing should also be avoided.
3.	Women should be aware of the decreased oxygen available for aerobic exercise during pregnancy. They should be encouraged to modify the intensity of their exercise according to maternal symptoms. Pregnant women should stop exercising when fatigued and not exercise to exhaustion. Weight-bearing exercises may, under some circumstances, be continued at intensities similar to those prior to pregnancy throughout pregnancy. Non-weight-bearing exercises, such as cycling or swimming, will minimize the risk of injury and facilitate the continuation of exercise during pregnancy.
4.	Morphologic changes in pregnancy should serve as a relative contraindication to types of exercise in which loss of balance could be detrimental to maternal or fetal well-being, especially in the third trimester. Further, any type of exercise involving the potential for even mild abdominal trauma should be avoided.
5.	Pregnancy requires an additional 300 kcal/d in order to maintain metabolic homeostasis. Thus, women who exercise during pregnancy should be particularly careful to ensure an adequate diet.
6.	Pregnant women who exercise in the first trimester should augment heat dissipation by ensuring adequate hydration, appropriate clothing, and optimal environmental surroundings during exercise.
7.	Many of the physiologic and morphologic changes of pregnancy persist four to six weeks postpartum. Thus, pre-pregnancy exercise routines should be resumed gradually, based upon a woman's physical capability.

* American College of Obstetricians and Gynecologists: *Exercise During Pregnancy and the Postpartum Period (Technical Bulletin #189)*. Washington, DC: ACOG, 1994.

FAQ #18

Question: Should I continue my aerobic workouts when I'm sick?

Answer: According to most sports medicine experts, the location of your symptoms can help determine whether it's safe for you to continue to exercise. In general, when your symptoms are experienced only above the neck (e.g., headache, runny or stuffy nose, scratchy throat, or sneezing), the infection is usually mild and won't be worsened by mild-to-moderate exercise. On the other hand, symptoms that occur below the neck or throughout the body (e.g., fever, chest cough, achy muscles, nausea, vomiting, or diarrhea) indicate that the infection may be more severe and requires rest. In fact, those symptoms are frequently associated with the flu, pneumonia, or some other potentially serious infection (viral or bacterial). If you do decide to exercise when you're not feeling your best, start at approximately 50 percent of your usual exercise intensity level. If, after about 10 minutes of exercising you feel no worse than before you started, you should gradually increase your intensity level—but stay well below your normal level of effort. If, however, the activity makes you feel worse, call it a day.

If you do decide to exercise when you're not feeling your best, start at approximately 50 percent of your usual exercise intensity level.

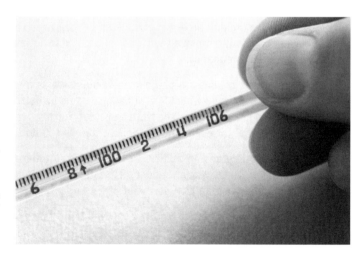

FAQ #19

Question: Having just begun to participate in a step aerobics class, do basic guidelines exist that I should follow so that I don't hurt myself?

Answer: To avoid placing yourself at risk for injury, you should adhere to the following bench-stepping (a.k.a., step aerobics) guidelines:

- Warm up for a few minutes by performing some arm movements and step patterns without the bench.

- To avoid knee injury, don't set the bench so high that you have to bend your knees more than 90 degrees at any point while stepping up.

- Stand no farther than a distance of one foot from the bench, to minimize stress on your Achilles tendon and the arch of your foot.

- When you step off the bench, place your foot on the floor toe first. Then, lower your heel to the floor before taking the next step—this practice will distribute your weight over the sole of your foot and reduce the level of stress placed on your foot.

- Avoid lunging movements. Those repeated, small leaps off the step increase the intensity of the workout, but also increase the impact stress on your joints.

- Look straight ahead. Staring down at your feet can cause neck and cervical back pain.

- Step exercising if you feel any pain in your joints. Be especially cautious if you've had previous knee pain or injury.

- Cool down after you exercise by walking or cycling for a few minutes. Then stretch.

FAQ #20

Question: Are saunas, hot tubs, or steam rooms dangerous for individuals suffering from hypertension (i.e., high blood pressure)?

Answer: Using saunas, hot tubs, or steam rooms can be dangerous for hypertensive individuals and those with heart disease. Surprisingly, however, it is not because the individual's blood pressure rises too high, but rather because it can drop to dangerously low levels. The basis for this dilemma is easier understood once the body's response to excess heat is examined.

The thermoregulatory mechanisms of the body cope with excess heat through two principal mechanisms: (1) sweating and (2) the redistribution of blood close to the surface of the skin so that heat can dissipate into the air. When an individual sweats, the moisture on the skin's surface evaporates, creating a cooling effect. In hot, humid environments, however, sweat does not readily evaporate. As a result, this evaporative cooling mechanism becomes ineffective and inefficient. In an effort to compensate, the peripheral arteries near the skin dilate, so that greater amounts of blood can be transferred to the skin's surface. This compensatory process is responsible for the characteristic "flushed look" individuals have when they become overheated. Redirecting blood flow to the peripheral arteries requires the heart to work harder.

In fact, the heat stress associated with using a sauna, hot tub, or steam room can be enough to cause the heart rate of an individual to nearly double in less than 10 minutes. In addition to performing its usual task of supplying the muscles and other vital organs (e.g., the brain) with sufficient amounts of blood, oxygen, and nutrients, the heart struggles to meet the demands for increased blood flow to the dilated peripheral arteries. The dilation of the peripheral arteries results in significantly less resistance to blood flow, and concomitantly, a dramatic drop in blood pressure (clinically referred to as hypotension).

Research has shown that heat stress from saunas, hot tubs, or steam rooms typically won't cause significant blood pressure changes in normotensive individuals. Hypertensive individuals on medication, however, may experience a rather sudden, dramatic drop in blood pressure. Such a hypotensive response can result in symptoms such as dizziness, light-headedness, and fainting. In order to compensate, the heart beats more rapidly, attempting to supply blood to all the areas of the body that require it. Left unchecked, this reaction can cause a complete collapse of the cardiovascular system. For a person with an already compromised cardiovascular system, the heart can beat at extremely rapid rates—potentially triggering a myocardial infarction (i.e., a heart attack) or cardiac arrest (cessation of the normal heartbeat). In summary, individuals who suffer from hypertension—or any other type of cardiac condition—should be advised to avoid using saunas, hot tubs, and steam rooms.

• •

FAQ #21

Question: Is it dangerous to run in subfreezing air?

Answer: Cold weather usually does not present a significant problem for most individuals who desire to exercise outdoors. For instance, cold air does not pose a particular danger to your respiratory passages. By the time inspired cold air reaches your lungs, the air is warmed to a temperature level that is safe for respiratory tissue. In fact, healthy individuals can breathe air at temperatures as low as -31°F without any harmful or detrimental effects. Breathing cold air, however, can be risky for individuals who suffer from asthma or angina. At-risk individuals, if cleared by their physicians to exercise in the cold, should wear ski masks or scarfs pulled loosely over their mouths—a preventive action that will help warm the inhaled air. Another, but very surprising, threat associated with exercising in subfreezing air is dehydration. When you exercise, you lose fluids by sweating and, particularly in the winter, by breathing. The dry winter air has to be warmed and moistened by the respiratory system. As you exhale, you lose water—when you "see" your breath, you're actually seeing tiny water droplets. In addition, urine production is stimulated by the cold. Consequently, as a precautionary measure, you should drink plenty of nonalcoholic beverages when exercising in the cold.

FAQ #22

Question: What prescriptive recommendations exist for minimizing the risk of injury or avoiding complications among beginning exercisers?

Answer: On occasion, deconditioned individuals or novice exercisers become very discouraged because of an undue level of muscular soreness or a musculoskeletal injury that results when they increase their exercise dosage too abruptly. The point to keep in mind is that exercise programs which require individuals to do too much (i.e., an intensity of > 90 percent $\dot{V}O_2$ max, a frequency of 5 days/week, or a duration of 45 minutes/session of training) offer the participant little or no additional improvement in aerobic fitness capacity ($\dot{V}O_2$ max) over those in which the demands placed on the exerciser are at an appropriate level. On the other hand, the incidence of orthopedic injury from undue demands increases substantially. Giving an adequate amount of attention to adequate warm-up, proper exercise shoes, and training on appropriate terrain (i.e., avoiding hard, uneven surfaces) or equipment (i.e., low-impact exercise modalities) should aid in decreasing attrition due to injury.

A recommended initial prescription (i.e., the first 6 to 8 weeks of training) for beginners is to exercise approximately 20-30 minutes every other day, at a perceived exertion of 4 (moderate) to 5 (somewhat strong) on a 10-point scale. Research, however, has shown that individuals can achieve similar training effects by performing three 10-minute bouts of moderate intensity exercise per day versus performing one "continuous" exercise bout of 30 minutes. Finally, participants should be counseled to discontinue exercising and seek medical advice if they experience certain warning signs or symptoms, including abnormal heart rhythms (palpitations), chest pain or pressure, or dizziness.

FAQ #23

Question: How can an individual distinguish cardiac chest pain from non-cardiac chest pain?

Answer: Usually, the main symptom of a cardiac chest pain (e.g., severe angina or a heart attack) is a heavy, squeezing, constricting, burning pain or discomfort occurring in the center of the chest. This pain may sometimes radiate down the left arm, across the left shoulder and upper back, or up to the neck and to the lower jaw. Anxiety, profuse sweating, nausea and vomiting, shortness of breath, and fainting may also be present. Fortunately, in most cases the pain or discomfort is severe enough to cause an individual to seek medical attention. In some instances, however, the pain lasts for only an hour or less and the individual mistakenly believes that the chest pain is simply due to indigestion or skeletal muscle spasms. The following questions can be useful in helping individuals to differentiate cardiac chest pain from non-cardiac chest pain:

- Does the pain/discomfort get better or worse when changing body position? Cardiac chest pain is not influenced by changes in body position.

- Is the pain/discomfort better or worse with respirations? Cardiac chest pain is not exacerbated by respiration.

- Is the pain/discomfort intense, dull, or knifelike? Cardiac chest pain is usually described as a dull ache or heaviness; it is seldom characterized as being sharp or stabbing.

- Is the pain/discomfort deep or close to the surface? Cardiac chest pain is deep, not superficial.

If you or a client experience sustained chest pain, with or without the other warning signs or symptoms described, seek immediate medical assistance—DO NOT WAIT TO SEE IF THE SYMPTOMS SUBSIDE. Individuals have nothing to lose (except perhaps a little time and money) if they go to the hospital on a false alarm, but they may very well save a life.

FAQ #24

Question: Given the high prevalence of back pain, do accepted general guidelines for treatment or prevention exist?

Answer: According to a task force of the Public Health Services Agency for Health Care Policy and Research, doctors, therapists, and patients, working together, can often resolve even the most stubborn cases of back pain. The task force developed the following new guidelines for back pain treatment:

- *Get medical attention immediately* for a severe back injury like a fall from a ladder or if a fever accompanies your back pain. If individuals experience loss of strength or numbness in their legs or if they have loss of bladder or bowel control, they should seek immediate medical attention.

- *Try at-home treatment* for a week or two before consulting a physician for mild to moderate episodes of back pain, but if symptoms appear to be worsening, contact a physician immediately.

- *After a muscle strain in the back,* it is recommended that an individual rest, but for no more than two or three days.

- *Take* over-the-counter pain killers.

- *Cold packs applied to the painful area* for five to ten minutes at a time are helpful within the first 48 hours after the injury. After the initial period, a heating pad, a warm whirlpool bath, or a hot shower may provide temporary relief.

- *Start your normal activities* and careful exercise as soon as possible.

Preventing back pain may be more effective and beneficial than treating it. Back specialists offer several suggestions for preventing back injuries and back pain including:

- *Don't smoke.* Studies show that individuals with severe back pain were more likely to be heavy smokers. Smoking reduces blood flow to the discs, possibly causing them to degenerate.

- *Lift properly.* The farther individuals hold or carry an object away from their bodies, the greater the potential for back injury. Individuals should bend from their knees and keep the object close to their bodies when they lift.

- *Don't sit for long periods.* Stand up at intervals, like when talking on the phone. When driving long distances, periodically stop and walk around. In an airplane, walk the aisles.

- *Use a good, stable chair.* It should have armrests, an anti-slide surface and back support. It also should be high enough so that the knees are slightly above the level of the hips.

- *Lose weight.* Carrying extra body weight, particularly in the abdominal region, can throw the body off balance, result in poor posture, and place added stress on the back.

- *Exercise regularly.* The muscles of the back, in combination with the spinal ligaments, provide the foundation of strength and support for the entire spinal column. Exercise increases the strength and efficiency of the trunk and lower back muscles. Consequently, the back is better able to withstand sudden movements and improper bending or lifting. Individuals should choose low-impact exercises (e.g., walking, stair climbing, cycling, etc.) that develop the back, trunk, and leg muscles without jarring the spine.

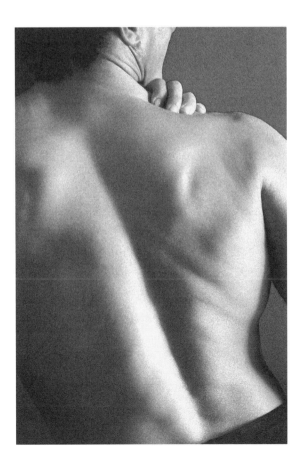

The muscles of the back, in combination with the spinal ligaments, provide the foundation of strength and support for the entire spinal column.

FAQ #25

Question: What are "Kegel" exercises and what are they designed to help?

Answer: Post-menopausal women are often advised to perform Kegel (the name of the gynecologist who invented it) exercise, which is designed to improve the tone of the muscles, ligaments, and fascia, collectively known as the pelvic floor. The pelvic floor serves several functions, including controlling urination and defecation, enhancing the sexual response to orgasm and providing support to the pelvic organs. Many women and men are unaware that their "pelvic floor" muscles can be strengthened just like their biceps or quadriceps.

Millions of women are affected by stress urinary incontinence. This condition is also common among men who have undergone prostate cancer surgery. Stress urinary incontinence is the involuntary loss of urine during physical exertion or activities such as laughing, sneezing, or coughing. Unfortunately, many women consider incontinence as an inevitable consequence of childbirth and aging, which it is not. Active women of all ages report experiencing incontinence. This situation can be particularly bothersome when it occurs during physical exertion. In fact, some women instead of seeking medical advice or beginning to perform a sound program involving the Kegel exercise, stop exercising, change their choice of activity, or begin wearing a protective pad. The point that these women fail to realize is that strengthening the pelvic floor muscles can provide them with much needed support and control.

Among the basic guidelines that women who want to perform Kegel exercise should adhere to are the following:

- Contract your anal sphincter as you would to stop unrinating or prevent a bowel movement. This action can be done while you're standing, sitting, or lying down.

- Hold the contraction for a count of four seconds, and then relax for four seconds. Don't tighten your abdominal, quadriceps, or gluteal muscles when performing this exercise.

- Perform the exercise at least twice a day.

It typically takes approximately eight weeks for Kegel exercises to result in a noticeable improvement in bladder control. Since no other exercise strengthens the pelvic floor muscles as effectively as these, many urinary incontinence experts recommend that all women athletes, including those without stress incontinence, perform Kegel exercises daily as a preventive measure.

• •

FAQ #26

Question: Please explain exactly what menopause is and how exercise can help control the symptoms associated with this condition?

Answer: The medical definition of menopause is cessation of menses for 12 months, caused when the ovaries stop making the hormones estrogen, progesterone, and testosterone. For most women, menopause simply marks the end of their reproductive years. While the average age for menopause is about 51, some women may experience it as early as their thirties or as late as their sixties. The symptoms of menopause include: hot flashes, night sweats, bladder and reproductive tract changes, insomnia, headaches, lethargy/fatigue, irritability, anxiety, depression, heart palpitations, and joint pain.

The good news is that a regular program of physical activity can help to manage many of the uncomfortable symptoms of menopause as well as the related health concerns, such as heart disease and osteoporosis. The mood-elevating, tension-relieving effects of aerobic exercise help reduce the depression and anxiety that often accompany menopause. Aerobic exercise also helps to promote the loss of abdominal fat—the place most women more readily gain weight during menopause. In addition, some research studies have shown that the acute increase in estrogen levels that follow an exercise bout coincide with an overall decrease in the severity of hot flashes. Strength training also helps by stimulating bones to retain the minerals that keep them dense and strong. This can prevent or delay the onset and progression of osteoporosis.

FAQ #27

Question: What general exercise recommendations and guidelines exist for asthmatics?

Answer: Most pulmonary experts suggest that the first step in formulating an exercise program for asthmatics is to evaluate how the individual's body responds to progressive exercise to volitional fatigue. The next step is to develop an exercise regimen that meets the individual's needs and interests. Among the guidelines that asthmatics should follow to ensure that their exercise programs are both safe and effective are:

- Select an exercise that raises the heart rate, increases the respiratory rate, and is relatively easy on the lungs. Swimming, for example, is one of the best tolerated exercise modalities by asthmatics.

- Avoid asthma triggers as much as possible. For example, asthmatics allergic to pollen should exercise indoors.

- Avoid exercising outdoors on either polluted or cold, dry days. Wear a mask or a scarf to warm and moisten the inspired air if the exercise bout must occur outside on a cold day. Whenever possible, exercise in warm, humid air.

- Perform specific breathing exercises to strengthen the lungs.

- Use ratings of perceived exertion in conjunction with target heart rate to regulate exercise intensity, since many of the asthma medications can alter an asthmatic's heart-rate response to exercise.

- Premedicate prior to exercising (within 30 minutes prior to engaging in activity).

- Keep an inhaler on hand while exercising.

- Avoid sudden, intense exercise for prolonged periods of time.

- Breathe through the nose as much as possible while exercising.

- Avoid hyperventilation by using a controlled breathing pattern.

FAQ #28

Question: What is plantar fascitis, and how should it be treated?

Answer: Plantar fascitis is an inflammation of the strong, fibrous tissue (i.e., plantar fascia) that runs along the bottom of the foot and connects the heel to the base of the toes. Along with the muscles and bones, the plantar fascia forms the arch of the foot. Plantar fascitis is a repetitive microtrauma overload injury. The diagnosis of plantar fascitis is most common among individuals involved in activities with repeated running and/or jumping. As an individual's foot bears weight, the arch flattens, overstretching the plantar fascia. Repeated flattening of the arch can inflame the plantar fascia, causing a nagging pain in the arch near the heel. The pain can be quite intense, particularly when walking or pressing down on that area. As a general rule, it is usually worse with the first few steps that an individual takes on a particular day. As the day progresses, the pain may lessen. Over the course of the day or with an increased amount of activity, however, it may actually worsen. Wearing shoes with poor arch support or a worn-out mid-sole can exacerbate matters. An effective treatment or rehabilitation program for plantar fascitis typically focuses on (1) managing the pain, (2) restoring flexibility to the ankle and the arch, (3) strengthening the intrinsic muscles in and around the foot, and (4) encouraging a gradual, progressive resumption of normal activities. Among the most common, effective treatments for plantar fascitis are ice, stretching, ultrasound, and orthotics (i.e., shoe inserts).

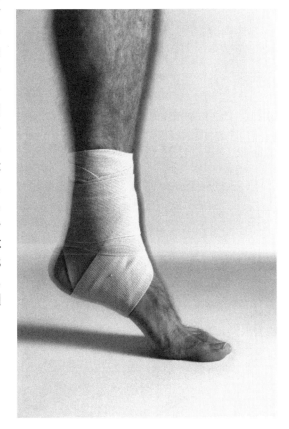

Plantar fascitis is a repetitive microtrauma overload injury.

FAQ #29

Question: How effective is exercise stress testing at screening individuals for underlying coronary heart disease (CHD)?

Answer: For an individual with chest pain of any type, an exercise stress test is a very effective diagnostic tool. Exercise stress test sensitivity (i.e., the test's ability to accurately identify individuals with CHD) is generally reported to be 55-70 percent.

$$\text{Sensitivity} = \frac{\text{True Positives}}{\text{True Positives} + \text{False Negatives}}$$

Where: True Positives = Individuals with CHD who are correctly identified

False Negatives = Individuals with CHD who are incorrectly identified as being disease free

In the same individual, the specificity of the test (i.e., the test's ability to correctly identify individuals who are free of CHD) is also highly accurate, with a specificity of 80-95 percent for men and 60-80 percent for women.

$$\text{Specificity} = \frac{\text{True Negatives}}{\text{True Negatives} + \text{False Positives}}$$

Where: True Negatives = Individuals without CHD who are correctly identified as being disease free

False Positives = Individuals without CHD who are incorrectly identified as having CHD

In symptom-free individuals who undergo an exercise stress test, however, the accuracy of the test declines. In this instance, both the sensitivity and specificity levels are low. A low sensitivity is especially concerning since it indicates that the test will not identify those with "silent" disease and, therefore, at risk for acute cardiovascular events. On the other hand, a low specificity level can lead to a significant number of false positive tests—a scenario that can create the problem of encouraging individuals who receive the inaccurate readings to unnecessarily undergo more extensive (and, often times, more costly) testing.

Research on the use of exercise stress testing as a screening tool has revealed three limitations. The first is that the majority of individuals who experience a cardiac event have negative exercise stress test results. Second, most individuals who test "positive" do not have significant coronary artery disease (i.e., greater than 50 percent stenosis angiographically). Despite these limitations, exercise stress testing can be used for symptomatic and asymptomatic individuals as an effective prognostic test for CHD. For example, clinical studies have shown that individuals tolerating more than 12 minutes of the Bruce test (a commonly used treadmill exercise protocol) and/or achieving a heart rate greater than 160 beats per minute had a one-year mortality rate of one percent regardless of the presence or absence of angiographic abnormalities. Furthermore, many health/fitness professionals have found that exercise stress testing has numerous useful applications, including quantifying fitness levels, determining a true maximum heart rate for exercise prescription, motivating clients, and assessing progress (or deterioration) over time.

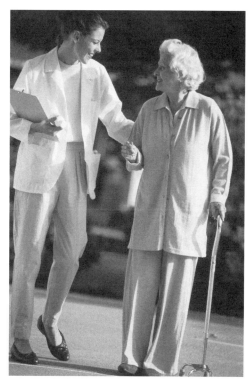

Finally, exercise testing is of little or no value in detecting mild-to-moderate coronary artery blockage (i.e., less than 70 percent occlusion). Yet, recent studies suggest that it is these lesions that are most likely to suddenly occlude. The likely result of this situation is a heart attack.

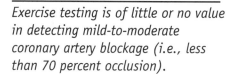

Exercise testing is of little or no value in detecting mild-to-moderate coronary artery blockage (i.e., less than 70 percent occlusion).

FAQ #30

Question: Is exercising on a stair climbing machine bad for the knees?

Answer: Despite intuitive beliefs to the contrary, exercising on an independent step-action, stair climbing machine is very safe for a person's knee joints. The contention that exercising on steppers might be bad for an individual's knees apparently stems from a concern over the forces generated at the knee during actual stair climbing (e.g., running stadium stairs). The estimated load factor on the knee while climbing actual stairs, for example, is approximately two times (while ascending) to seven times (while descending) an individual's body weight. On the other hand, research has shown that the orthopedic loads on the body while exercising on an independent step-action stair climbing machine are just slightly greater than body weight (approximately 1.2 times—a level comparable to walking).

The functional movement patterns involved in exercising on a stair climbing machine also help to protect an individual's knees. Biomechanical assessments of individuals involving electromyography and force diagrams have indicated that anterior strain (i.e., shear stress) on the knee is greatly reduced while exercising on an independent step-action stepper. This reduction in knee strain is a direct result of the axial (central) orientation of the applied load and the muscular co-contraction of the quadriceps and hamstrings that occur during the exercise. These factors substantially reduce an individual's risk of experiencing patellofemoral discomfort during and/or following a stair climbing workout. In short, a major benefit of exercising on a stair climbing machine is that it duplicates running up a hill or stadium stairs, but without all the pounding to the joints and muscles.

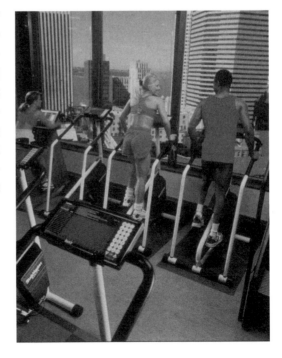

Exercising on an independent step-action, stair climbing machine has been found to be very safe for a person's knee joints.

FAQ #31

Question: What effect, if any, does exercising in air pollution have on my workout performance?

Answer: A by-product of extremely complex chemical reactions, air pollution can negatively impact an individual's aerobic exercise capacity in several ways. The magnitude of air pollution's effect is at least partly related to the ability of pollutants (e.g., carbon monoxide, ozone, sulfur dioxide, etc.) to infiltrate your respiratory system.

When you are not engaged in physical activity, your respiratory tract serves as both the major route of infiltration for air pollutants and the major barrier to their penetration. For example, during normal inspiration, the mucous membranes in the nose are very effective in removing large particulate matter and highly soluble gases from the air that reach the lungs. On the other hand, during aerobic exercise you tend to breathe through your mouth, the natural air filtration process of the body becomes less efficient, resulting in more pollutants reaching the lungs. Once in the lungs, many of these pollutants subsequently diffuse into the bloodstream and circulate through the body.

Since the respiratory tract is the largest surface area of the body to come in contact with air pollutants, many of the adverse effects of air pollution occur in that region. Among the many negative physiologic effects of air pollution are the following:

- Bronchial vasoconstriction (i.e., the airway openings become smaller), occurs which results in increased airway resistance.

- The lungs lose some of their diffusing surface area either as a result of destruction of the alveoli (i.e., the functional units of the lung) or as a by-product of an increased level of mucus secretion.

- Oxygen transport capacity is reduced. Less oxygen enters the bloodstream (via the pulmonary system), resulting in an inadequate supply of oxygenated blood to the exercising muscles.

The net result is that these negative physiologic effects of air pollution can cause a substantial decrease in your physical performance.

FAQ #32

Question: How safe is aerobic dance as an exercise activity?

Answer: Several studies have found that a substantial number of participants in aerobic dance suffer injuries of one form or another. Injury rates for participants have been estimated to be about one injury for every 100 hours of aerobic dancing, and for instructors, about one per 400 hours.

Questions arise regarding what kinds of injuries are associated with aerobic dance and whether the physical and emotional benefits of aerobic dance outweigh the risks of being injured. Most aerobic dance injuries tend to involve the lower extremities (about 80 percent of all such injuries) and result from excessive physical trauma. Classified as either acute (i.e., stress is applied too abruptly to tissues not prepared to handle them) or overuse (i.e., repeated stresses are applied over time to tissues, causing microscopic damage to the tissues, which never get the opportunity to heal), aerobic dance injuries range from mild muscle pulls and strains, ankle sprains, inflamed tendons, heel spurs, and knee pain to stress fractures.

Research studies suggest that the three most prevalent risk factors for aerobic dancing are stressing the body too often (i.e., exercising more than three times per week), wearing improper shoes, and exercising on non-resilient surfaces. Research has also found that aerobic dance participants are at risk regardless of whether they engage in high-impact (i.e., ballistic jumping and dancing on the balls of the feet) or low-impact (at least one foot remains in contact with the ground at all times) aerobics. While the risks appear to be greater during high-impact aerobics because of the orthopedic trauma associated with ballistic stresses, low-impact aerobic dancing also involves an increased potential for injury because its often exaggerated movements can place biomechanically unnatural stress on the knees, ankles, and lower back.

Do the benefits of aerobic dancing outweigh its risks? In most cases, they do—particularly when the participant takes a sensible approach to exercising . . . doesn't try to do too much too soon . . . builds up gradually in both intensity and duration . . . prepares the body for the stresses imposed by aerobic dancing (e.g., strengthen the muscles supporting the ligaments involved in the exercise) . . . warms up and stretches before exercising . . . and learns and practices biomechanically correct techniques and movements for the exercise. While, by definition, exercise involves stress to your body and without such stress your body would not make the physiological adaptations that enable you to improve your fitness level, it is neither sensible nor productive to push your body beyond the limits it can reasonably sustain.

Aerobic dancing has been shown to produce a demonstrable training effect when participants adhere to appropriate levels of intensity, frequency, and duration. The risk of injury associated with aerobic dance can never be entirely eliminated, but most of the potential problems can be avoided simply by using "common sense" and listening to your body's important warning signals (e.g., pain, discomfort, excessive fatigue, etc.).

• •

FAQ #33

Question: Can exercise help arthritis sufferers?

Answer: Absolutely. A number of studies have shown that low-impact exercise (e.g., swimming, cycling, stair climbing, walking, etc.) is beneficial for individuals with arthritis—particularly those with rheumatoid arthritis and osteoarthritis, the two most common forms of this painful condition. Even those people who have to undertake an extended bout of rest because of experiencing a severe arthritis flare-up are encouraged to keep their joints moving as much as possible.

Among the documented benefits of sound exercise for arthritis sufferers are an improvement in muscle strength, an enhanced level of stamina, and an increased ability of the body's joints to move more freely, with less swelling and pain. By strengthening the shock-absorbing muscles and ligaments and tendons around the joints, exercise is able to take some of the pressure off those joints. Furthermore, exercise has been shown to provide some arthritis sufferers with an enhanced level of energy that, in turn, gives these individuals a renewed sense of hope and control over the quality of their lives.

The key factor in any arthritis exercise program should be to increase joint flexibility, muscular strength, and overall stamina—without stressing the body's joints. High-impact activities or those activities that involve sudden twisting movements (e.g., racquetball, basketball, etc.) should be avoided. Strengthening exercises, low-impact or non-impact aerobic exercise and exercises designed to take any joint in the body slowly and safely through a pain-free range of motion are recommended.

FAQ #34

Question: What basic steps can I take to minimize the risks associated with exercising?

Answer: Unfortunately, no human endeavor is totally free of risk—including exercise. The risks of exercise, however, can be minimized by adhering to certain principles and guidelines. The first step is to ensure that you are medically safe to exercise. This process involves seeing a physician and undergoing a physical examination and evaluation *before* you initiate your exercise program. The extent of your evaluation depends on your age, health status, and the anticipated exercise intensity. For example, all older asymptomatic individuals (males 40 plus, females 50 plus) or at high risk (e.g., having one or more risk factors, including smoking, hypertension, high blood cholesterol, obesity, stress, family history of medical problems, diabetes) should undergo a physician-supervised, graded exercise test. Healthy individuals under age 40 for men and 50 for women are usually cleared for exercise upon completing a medical/health status questionnaire, if the answers don't reveal any possible contraindications to exercise.

The next step is to develop a sound exercise program based on scientifically documented information. Such a program should involve starting at an intensity appropriate for you and then progressing gradually to a point where your body must respond to increasingly higher physical demands. The temptation to do too much too soon should be avoided. Moderation is essential. The point to remember is that a major cause of musculoskeletal injuries is overuse—placing demands on your body that your body simply is not designed to handle. A sound exercise program always includes provisions for stretching the major joints of your body before and after exercising. It also ensures that you get proper rest (sleep). Rest enables you to better recover from the demands placed on your body by exercising.

The final step is to listen to your body. You should respond accordingly to common exercise termination signals (e.g., dizziness, lightheadedness, abnormal heart beats, pain or pressure in your chest, musculoskeletal trauma, prolonged fatigue, etc.). These signals are your body's way of telling you that something is amiss and that you must decrease the level of stress to which you are subjecting your body.

FAQ #35

Question: Do sports rubs and liniments, such as Ben-Gay® or Icy Hot®, help promote tissue healing?

Answer: Sports cremes and rubs are popular, convenient methods of producing soothing feelings of warmth or cold in the muscles. Their effect, however, is only superficial. The active ingredients in the various sports rubs stimulate sensory nerve endings in the skin to produce sensations of heat or cold that temporarily mask the pain and the discomfort of muscular soreness. On one hand, the massaging action typically associated with the application of sports rubs may increase localized blood flow and possibly cause the muscles to relax. On the other hand, since the heating or cooling action is artificial, sports rubs do little or nothing to promote tissue healing.

• • • • • • • • • • • • • • • • • • • •

FAQ 36

Question: I'm somewhat confused by the wide array of advertisements in both my local newspaper and on television for aerobic-type exercise machines. How can I know which machine would be best for me?

Answer: Unfortunately, many of the exercise machines/devices marketed on television are less than advertised. Not only are many of them shoddily built, they also have a tendency to subject users to an undue risk of injury because of their unsafe design. Essentially, you have two logical choices when it comes to selecting aerobic exercise equipment. First, you can contact one of the premier health, wellness and fitness organizations in the country to ask them for advice, for example, either the American Council on Exercise (1-800-529-8227) or the American College of Sports Medicine (1-317-637-9200). Second, if you belong to a local health club, YMCA, or JCC, you should try out the aerobic exercise equipment that this particular facility has to offer. Provided you ensure that the tryout period lasts for at least a few weeks, your body will let you know if it likes your choice of exercise machines.

FAQ #37

Question: What is a "runner's high" and what factors are responsible for it?

Answer: The runner's high has been described as a feeling of well-being and, in some instances, euphoria that many runners experience during long-distance runs. The exact mechanisms responsible for the phenomenon are unknown.

Such a high is most often reported by experienced runners who regularly run long distances and who try to mentally dissociate while running. Their minds are preoccupied with various thoughts, the majority of which have nothing to do with running. Such diversions allow the runner to escape from the discomfort and pain that often accompany running. Running—with its rhythmic pace and controlled breathing pattern—can be compared with meditation. Elite runners, however, like to tune in to their body's signals and use these signals to develop strategies during a race. They would view the mental dissociation of the runner's high as being detrimental to their optimum race performance.

Research suggests that the runner's high may have a physiological basis. The stress of running may increase the body's blood level of endorphins (chemical compounds produced by the pituitary gland and other areas of the body). Endorphins are thought to have a morphine-like effect that masks pain and produces feelings of euphoria.

Research on endorphins, however, has been mixed. Studies that correlate the blood level of endorphins with subjective feelings may be misleading, since no one has been able to objectively describe exactly how the runner's high feels. In addition, the placebo effect of anticipating a high could strongly influence the results of a study by producing artificial correlations. Perhaps, most importantly, the blood level of endorphins does not necessarily reflect what is happening in the brain because the blood-brain barrier insulates the brain from the circulatory system. In fact, researchers, who have chemically blocked the effects of endorphins, have found that the runner's high still occurred, suggesting that endorphins might not be involved.

A connection between compulsive runners and the runner's high may exist. These runners possess a need to run to make it through the day. It could be that the effect of such a "fix" is multifaceted. One part may satisfy the psychological compulsion to run, another may provide a mental diversion from stressful events of the day, and yet another may ease the physical craving for the endorphin effect. If any part is missing, the high may not occur. As a result, nonaddicted or novice runners often may not experience the so-called runner's high.

. . . .

FAQ #38

Question: How important are the warm-up and cool-down portions of a workout?

Answer: Warm-up and cool-down activities should be an essential part of all exercise programs. The purpose of warm-up activities is to prepare the body, especially the cardiovascular and musculoskeletal systems, for the conditioning or stimulus phase of the exercise session. Our experience suggests that the ideal warm-up for any endurance activity is that activity—only at a lower intensity. Hence, participants who engage in brisk walking during the endurance phase of their workout should conclude the warm-up period with slow walking. The cool-down phase assures that venous return to the heart is maintained in the face of significant amounts of blood going to the previously working muscles. Light aerobic endurance activities, coupled with stretching activities, provide the fundamental basis for both the warm-up and cool-down phases. The length of the warm-up and cool-down periods depends on several factors, including the type of activity engaged in during the conditioning period, the intensity of those activities, and the age and fitness level of the participant. In general, the warm-up and cool-down phases should last approximately five to ten minutes each. If the individual has less time available to work out than usual, it is recommended that the time allotted for the conditioning phase of the workout be reduced, while retaining sufficient time for both the warm-up and cool-down phases.

FAQ #39

Question: Does using hand and ankle weights improve the quality of an aerobic workout?

Answer: Research has shown that using small weights (i.e., one to five pounds) increases the heart rate, the oxygen uptake, and the total number of calories expended during an aerobic activity. The magnitude of the increase is typically only 5-10 percent—a value that is much less than the claims made by most advocates of using hand or ankle weights. Individuals can easily achieve similar increases in energy output by exercising a little longer or at a slightly higher level of intensity. The following factors should be considered by individuals who are contemplating using hand or ankle weights:

- Added weights can increase the risk of orthopedic injury during exercise—particularly activities such as traditional aerobic dance or running.

- Individuals with hypertension (i.e., high blood pressure) or coronary heart disease should use caution when exercising with supplemental weights (particularly hand weights), because the use of such devices during aerobic exercise can significantly tax the cardiovascular system.

- Added weights, while exercising aerobically, can decrease an individual's level of mechanical efficiency, thereby causing fatigue to occur more quickly.

For most individuals, the issue of whether to use supplemental weights during exercise is fairly straightforward—the drawbacks of wearing hand and/or ankle weights during aerobic workouts outweigh any potential benefits.

FAQ #40

Question: Is heavy sweating while engaging in physical activity a dangerous sign?

Answer: If an individual is in good physical condition, chronic heavy sweating should not be a health concern. Most inactive people sweat anywhere from a negligible amount to two quarts per day, but heat and physical exertion can increase this amount to as much as five to 10 quarts. Age, race, gender, fitness level, and sensitivity to heat also affect the amount an individual sweats. A few individuals suffer from hyperhidrosis (a genetic condition) which causes them to perspire so profusely that their clothing can become drenched within several minutes of light activity. This condition is generally treated with topical antiperspirants. Although individuals can have their sweat glands removed, such surgery is rarely recommended because of the subsequent scarring that typically occurs. On the other hand, if an individual who normally does not sweat much suddenly starts to do so, it may be due to fever and illness or, in the case of women, the onset of menopause. Sweating can, however, be dangerous if it leads to dehydration. The best approach for a person to take is to drink plenty of fluids (irrespective of thirst) before, during, and after exercise.

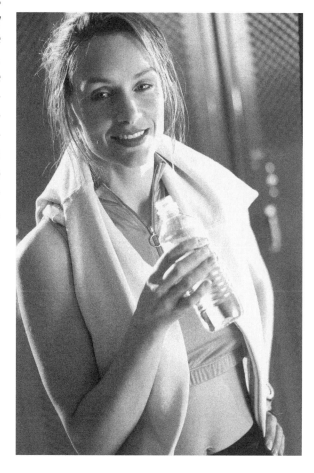

The best approach for a person to take with regard to hydration is to drink plenty of fluids (irrespective of thirst) before, during, and after exercise.

FAQ #41

Question: Should physically active women wear sports bras?

Answer: According to available sports science research, more than half of all physically active women experience some form of breast discomfort while exercising. In this regard, a number of experts have suggested that some women, particularly large-breasted individuals, may benefit from wearing sports bras while exercising. Unfortunately, many "so-called" sports bras aren't any better than regular model bras. The following are among the most important considerations when shopping for a sports bra:

- Keep in mind that sports bras come in two basic types—those that compress the breasts and those that encapsulate each breast. A woman should try on both types to find which is best for her.

- Simulate the motions of the physical activity you plan to engage in when trying on the bra.

- Select the bra with either seamless cups or seams that don't cross the nipple area.

- Avoid models with hooks, fasteners, or rough seams that may cause chaffing of the skin.

- Make sure the bands at the top and bottom of the bra are slightly elastic and wide enough to control bouncing and to prevent the bra from riding up.

- Be sure the straps of the bra do not dig into the shoulders.

FAQ #42

Question: Is running downhill more stressful on the knees than running uphill?

Answer: Contrary to popular opinion, running downhill is much more stressful on the joints and muscles in your feet and legs than running uphill. As you go down a hill, because you tend to speed up and lengthen your stride, the level of the impact force with the ground that your body is subjected to increases. When you jog on level terrain, your feet strike the ground with forces equivalent to approximately three times your body weight. However, the impact forces when running downhill can be as high as seven times your body weight. In addition, because your muscles simultaneously "tense-up" and lengthen (i.e., contract eccentrically) when you run downhill, your risk of experiencing delayed-onset muscle soreness is significantly increased. Furthermore, individuals tend to greatly alter their running mechanics when going downhill. The resultant distortion in gait pattern can lead to the development of a condition known as patellofemoral syndrome (i.e., "runner's knee")—pain or discomfort behind the kneecap. To avoid exposing yourself to an undue risk of injury, never run straight down a steep hill. Walk or run down such hills in a zigzag pattern, leaning slightly forward, and keeping your knees bent.

• • • • • • • • • • • • • • • • • • • •

FAQ #43

Question: I see some cyclists with their seats set high and others with their seats set low. Is there an optimal seat adjustment so I won't fatigue so easily?

Answer: Whether you're riding an stationary cycle or an outdoor bicycle, you should adjust your seat height so that a slight bend exists at the knee joint when your leg is fully extended with your foot on the pedal. If your seat is set too low, your quadriceps muscles will tend to fatigue more easily, thereby limiting your performance.

FAQ #44

Question: Does a relatively practical method exist for assessing a runner's aerobic fitness level?

Answer: Two of the most widely used running tests for assessing aerobic fitness are the Cooper 12-minute walk-run test and the 1.5-mile run test for time. The primary performance-related goal for an individual who takes the 12-minute walk-run test is to cover the greatest amount of distance in the allotted time period. While in the case of the 1.5-mile run test, the individual being tested attempts to run the distance in as short a period of time as possible. For both of these running tests, normative data are available to provide a reasonably accurate estimate of the aerobic fitness level of the individual who has been tested (refer to Tables 3 and 4). One of the most positive features of these tests is that they are very easy to administer. On the other hand, such performance-based tests have a few substantial limitations. For one thing, an individual's level of motivation and pacing ability can have a profound impact on that person's test results. Of greater potential importance, a certain degree of risk exists during such testing due to the fact that in both tests individuals are encouraged to put forth a maximal effort.

Key For Tables #3 & #4		
S	=	Superior
E	=	Excellent
G	=	Good
F	=	Fair
P	=	Poor
VP	=	Very Poor

Table 3. Aerobic Power Tests (Men)

%	MAX $\dot{V}O_2$ (ml/kg/ min)	12 MIN Run Distance (miles)	1.5 Mile Run (time)	MAX $\dot{V}O_2$ (ml/kg/ min)	12 MIN Run Distance (miles)	1.5 Mile Run (time)	Rating
	AGE 20-29			**Age 30-39**			
99	58.79	1.94	7:29	58.86	1.89	7:11	S
95	53.97	1.81	8:13	52.53	1.77	8:44	
90	51.35	1.74	9:09	50.36	1.71	9:30	E
85	49.64	1.69	9:45	48.20	1.65	10:16	
80	48.20	1.65	10:16	46.75	1.61	10:47	
75	46.99	1.62	10:42	45.31	1.57	11:18	G
70	46.75	1.61	10:47	44.59	1.55	11:34	
65	45.31	1.57	11:18	43.87	1.53	11:49	
60	44.23	1.54	11:41	42.42	1.49	12:20	
55	43.87	1.53	11:49	41.58	1.47	12:38	F
50	42.49	1.50	12:18	40.98	1.45	12:51	
45	42.42	1.49	12:20	39.53	1.41	13:22	
40	40.98	1.45	12:51	38.86	1.39	13:36	
35	40.26	1.43	13:06	38.09	1.37	13:53	P
30	39.53	1.41	13:22	37.37	1.35	14.08	
25	38.09	1.37	13:53	36.65	1.33	14:24	
20	37.13	1.34	14:13	35.35	1.29	14:52	
15	36.65	1.33	14:24	34.00	1.25	15:20	VP
10	34.48	1.27	15:10	32.53	1.21	15:52	
5	31.57	1.19	61:12	30.87	1.17	16:27	
1	27.09	1.06	14:48	26.54	1.13	18:00	
	N=1,675			N=7,094			

*Max $\dot{V}O2$ is a laboratory-derived measure that is generally considered to be the best indicator of an individual's level of aerobic capacity.

Table 3. Aerobic Power Tests (Men)–Continued.

%	Age 40-49 MAX $\dot{V}O_2$ (ml/kg/min)	12 Min Run Distance (miles)	1.5 Mile Run (time)	Age 50-59 MAX $\dot{V}O_2$ (ml/kg/min)	12 Min Run Distance (miles)	1.5 Mile Run (time)	Age 60+ MAX $\dot{V}O_2$ (ml/kg/min)	12 Min Run Distance (miles)	1.5 Mile Run (time)	Rating
99	55.42	1.85	7:42	52.53	1.77	8:44	50.39	1.71	9:30 S	S
95	50.36	1.71	9:30	47.11	1.62	10:40	45.21	1.57	11:20	
90	48.20	1.65	10:16	45.31	1.57	11:18	42.46	1.49	12:20	
85	45.31	1.57	11:18	42.42	1.49	12:20	39.53	1.41	13:22	E
80	44.11	1.54	11:44	40.98	1.45	12:51	38.09	1.37	13:53 E	
75	443.89	1.53	11:49	39.53	1.41	13:22	36.65	1.30	14:24	
70	41.75	1.47	12:34	38.45	1.38	13:45	35.30	1.29	14:53	G
65	40.98	1.45	12:51	37.61	1.35	14:03	39.29	1.26	15:19	
60	39.89	1.42	13:14	36.65	1.33	14:24	33.59	1.24	15:29 G	
55	39.53	1.41	13:22	36.10	1.31	14:40	32.39	1.21	15:55	
50	38.09	1.37	13:53	35.20	1.29	14:55	31.83	1.19	16:07	F
45	37.37	1.35	14:08	34.12	1.26	15:08	30.87	1.17	16:27	
40	36.68	1.33	14:29	33.76	1.25	15:26	30.15	1.15	16:43 F	
35	35.56	1.30	14:47	32.48	1.22	15:53	29.43	1.13	16:58	
30	35.13	1.29	14:56	32.31	1.21	15:57	28.70	1.11	17:14	P
25	33.76	1.25	15:26	31.06	1.17	16:23	27.89	1.08	17:32	
20	33.04	1.23	15:41	30.15	1.15	16:43	26.54	1.05	18:00 P	
15	32.31	1.21	15:57	29.43	1.13	16:58	25.09	1.01	18:31	
10	30.85	1.17	16:28	27.98	1.09	17:29	23.05	.95	19:15	VP
5	28.29	1.10	17:23	25.09	1.01	18:31	20.76	.89	20:04 VP	
1	24.15	.98	18:51	22.06	.92	19:36	18.28	.82	20:57	
	N=6,837			N=3,808			N=1,005			

Table 4. Aerobic Power Tests (Women)

%	Age 20-29			Age 30-39			Rating
	MAX $\dot{V}O_2$ (ml/kg/ min)	12 Min Run Distance (miles)	1.5 Mile Run (time)	MAX $\dot{V}O_2$ (ml/kg/ min)	12 Min Run Distance (miles)	1.5 Mile Run (time)	
99	53.03	1.78	8:33	48.73	1.66	10:05	S
95	46.75	1.61	10:47	43.87	1.53	11:49	
90	44.15	1.54	11:43	40.98	1.45	12:51	E
85	42.42	1.49	12:20	40.26	1.43	13.06	
80	40.98	1.45	12:51	38.57	1.38	13:43	
75	39.53	1.41	13:22	37.37	1.35	14:08	G
70	38.09	1.37	13:53	36.65	1.33	14:24	
65	37.37	1.35	14:08	35.44	1.29	14:50	
60	36.65	1.33	14:24	34.60	1.27	15:08	
55	36.14	1.31	14:35	33.85	1.26	15:20	F
50	35.20	1.29	14:55	33.76	1.25	15:26	
45	34.48	1.27	15:10	32.41	1.22	15:47	
40	33.76	1.25	15:26	32.31	1.21	15:57	
35	32.72	1.22	15:48	31.09	1.17	16:23	P
30	32.31	1.21	15:57	30.51	1.16	16:35	
25	30.94	1.17	16:26	29.93	1.13	16:58	
20	30.63	1.16	16:33	28.70	1.11	17:14	
15	29.43	1.13	16:58	27.98	1.09	17:29	VP
10	28.39	1.10	17:21	26.54	1.05	18:00	
5	25.89	1.03	18:14	25.09	1.01	18:31	
1	22.57	.94	19:25	22.49	.93	19:27	
	N=764			N=2,049			

* Max $\dot{V}O_2$ is a laboratory-derived measure that is generally considered to be the best indicator of an individual's level of aerobic capacity.

Table 4. Aerobic Power Tests (Women)-Continued.

%	MAX $\dot{V}O_2$ (ml/kg/ min)	12 Min Run Distance (miles)	1.5 Mile Run (time)	MAX $\dot{V}O_2$ (ml/kg/ min)	12 Min Run Distance (miles)	1.5 Mile Run (time)	MAX $\dot{V}O_2$ (ml/kg/ min)	12 Min Run Distance (miles)	1.5 Mile Run (time)	Rating
	Age 40-49			**Age 50-59**			**Age 60+**			
99	46.75	1.61	10:47	42.04	1.48	12:28	44.47	1.55	11:36	S
95	40.98	1.45	12:51	36.81	1.33	14:20	37.46	1.35	14:06	
90	39.53	1.41	13:22	35.20	1.29	14:55	35.20	1.29	14:55	E
85	37.49	1.35	14:06	33.59	1.24	15:29	32.31	1.21	15:57	
80	36.28	1.32	14:31	32.31	1.21	15:57	31.23	1.18	16:20	
75	335.11	1.29	14:57	39.90	1.20	16:05	30.87	1.17	16:27	G
70	33.76	1.25	15:16	30.87	1.17	16:27	29.43	1.13	16:58	
65	33.04	1.23	15:41	29.76	1.14	16:51	27.98	1.09	17:29	
60	32.31	1.21	15:57	29.43	1.13	16:58	27.21	1.07	17:46	
55	31.59	1.19	16:12	28.70	1.11	17:14	26.54	1.05	18:00	F
50	30.87	1.17	16:27	28.22	1.10	17:24	25.82	1.03	18:16	
45	30.58	1.16	16:34	27.98	1.09	17:29	25.09	1.01	18:31	
40	29.45	1.13	16:58	26.85	1.06	17:55	24.49	.99	18:44	
35	29.43	1.12	16:59	26.13	1.04	18:09	24.03	.98	18:54	P
30	28.25	1.10	17:24	25.48	1.02	18:23	23.80	.97	18:59	
25	27.98	1.09	17:29	25.09	1.01	18:31	23.65	.97	19:02	
20	26.54	1.05	18:00	24.25	.98	18:49	22.78	.94	19:21	
15	25.57	1.02	18:21	23.65	.97	19:02	22.21	.93	19:33	VP
10	25.09	1.01	18:31	22.33	.93	19:30	20.76	.89	20:04	
5	23.53	.96	19:05	21.10	.90	19:57	19.68	.86	20:23	
1	20.76	.89	20:04	18.74	.83	20:47	17.87	.81	21:06	
	N=1,630			N=878			N=202			

FAQ #45

Question: How should a first-time marathoner train to run a marathon?

Answer: The key is to determine what level of exposure to stress your body can handle to elicit the degree of adaptation that will enable you to successfully complete a marathon. In simple terms, how far, how fast, and how much should you train?

Before attempting to answer the fundamental training question of how far, how fast, and how much, you need to carefully consider the nature of a marathon. The marathon is an endurance event—not a speed undertaking. Endurance is a basic component of fitness that should be gradually developed through aerobic training. As has been previously discussed, aerobic training for running involves moving at a pace that (while stressful) will allow your body's requirements for oxygen to be fulfilled through respiration (i.e., breathing) over the duration of the run.

Unfortunately, no magic formula exists concerning how to train to complete a marathon. Over the years, a number of exercise scientists have unsuccessfully attempted to identify a mileage/pace equation for training for a marathon that can be applied to particular types or groups of individuals. The results of these efforts have been equivocal at best. The bottom line is that no perfect equation for marathon training exists. What does appear to matter most, however, are the total miles you run and the pace at which you run each mile. All other factors being equal, marathon training involves "putting in the miles." Exactly how many miles you put in each week depends on several factors (e.g., whom you talk to, your pre-training level of fitness, etc.). *Most references on the subject suggest a minimum of 60-70 miles per week for several months preceding the marathon event.* Obviously, how you distribute the miles (i.e., how long each particular run is) and how fast you run each mile are also matters that have to be addressed in a considered manner. Developing a specific training schedule can be a by-product of several sources (e.g., advice from an exercise specialist, the result of a trial-and-error approach on your part, or a sample plan gleaned from one of the numerous references on marathon training which are currently available on the market). Two common elements seem to apply to all successful marathon conditioning regimens: training regularly (i.e., almost every day) and training smart (i.e., alternate hard and easy workout days).

FAQ #46

Question: What basic guidelines should a "first-time" treadmill use follow?

Answer: Like any other exercise tool, using a treadmill safely and effectively requires that you follow certain steps and precautions. Regardless of whether or not you are an experienced treadmill user, you should adhere to the following guidelines:

- Get on the treadmill and straddle the belt by standing on the platform.

- Never turn the belt on while you're standing on it.

- Turn the belt on and look down at the belt to see how fast it is moving. Make sure it is going at a relatively slow speed.

- Hold on to either the side or the front handrails (depending on the type of treadmill you're using) before you step on to the moving belt.

- Start walking slowly to get the feel of exercising on the particular surface of the treadmill. Your body has to get acclimated to a different sense of balance on the treadmill.

- Warm up for a few minutes at a relatively slow speed to get accustomed to exercising on the treadmill. Then, gradually increase your speed to the rate you prefer. In the last few minutes of your workout, gradually decrease the rate of speed as a warm-down.

- While exercising, always look forward. Never look behind you or to the side because it tends to throw your balance off. If you must turn to talk to someone, hold on to a handrail.

- As a general rule, don't walk or run backwards on a treadmill.

- If while you're exercising you start to lose your balance, hold on to a handrail and step off. Don't try to stop the treadmill while you're off balance.

- Don't make major, sudden changes in speed while you're exercising. Do it gradually. More often than not, a higher level of speed can be much more difficult than the average individual believes it's going to be.

- When you decide to stop exercising, press the stop button, but continue to walk until the treadmill comes to a complete stop. Stay on the treadmill and hold on to the handrails for 30 to 60 seconds before you actually get off, in order to restore your sense of equilibrium, balance, and stability.

• •

FAQ #47

Question: I recently moved to Durango, Colorado from Las Vegas, Nevada. Is it my imagination or am I working harder when I jog in my new environment?

Answer: In a word, yes. You moved from a city relatively close to sea level to a town considerably higher in altitude. Your body can feel the difference and is responding accordingly. As you increase the altitude at which you are exercising, the barometric pressure decreases. Although the percentage of oxygen in the air stays fairly constant as the altitude increases, the amount of hemoglobin saturated with oxygen in your blood falls. Because the decrease in barometric pressure has a negative effect on the partial pressure of oxygen in the air you inspire, your level of hemoglobin saturation is also lowered. The net result is that since less oxygen is carried by your arterial blood, the amount of oxygen available at the cellular level is reduced. In turn, your level of maximal oxygen uptake ($\dot{V}O2$ max) and your physical working capacity (PWC) are reduced (relative to the increase in altitude). In an attempt to compensate for these changes, your body undergoes several adaptive responses. Submaximal heart rate, cardiac output, and pulmonary ventilation increase. To a point, your body can achieve the same level of submaximal performance, but has to work much harder to do so.

FAQ #48

Question: How much improvement in aerobic capacity can a person typically expect to experience, and how long does it take?

Answer: Increases in cardiorespiratory fitness with exercise training generally show a positive correlation to the frequency, intensity, and duration of exercise. The amount of improvement in aerobic capacity (i.e., $\dot{V}O2$ max) that can be expected from training is very individualized and is inversely related to each individual's level of fitness. In other words, the more fit an individual is the smaller the degree of improvement in $\dot{V}O2$ max associated with training. For example, an untrained individual may experience approximately a 25 percent increase in $\dot{V}O2$ max after roughly 8 to 12 weeks of conditioning. A trained individual, on the other hand, may experience only a five percent improvement over the same period of time.

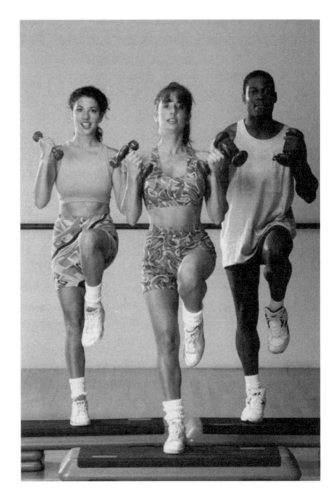

The amount of improvement in aerobic capacity (i.e., VO2 max) that can be expected from training is very individualized and is inversely related to each individual's level of fitness.

FAQ #49

Question: How can I tell how aerobically fit I am?

Answer: Because the procedures which can be used to assess aerobic fitness vary considerably in their ease of administration, cost, and degree of accuracy, you need to give careful consideration to your choices. The most widely accepted measure of aerobic fitness is your level of maximal oxygen uptake ($\dot{V}O_2$ max). A reflection of the greatest rate at which you can consume oxygen while exercising, $\dot{V}O_2$ max can be assessed in either a laboratory or a non-laboratory setting. When conducted in a laboratory, $\dot{V}O_2$ max testing usually involves the direct measurement of the gases you expire while exercising during either a maximal or near-maximal effort. An analysis of the volume of expired air and oxygen and carbon dioxide levels provides a very accurate measurement of $\dot{V}O2$ max. It is also possible to estimate your $\dot{V}O2$ max level in a laboratory setting without collecting gases by identifying the highest work load you can achieve while exercising before the onset of undue fatigue. In a non-laboratory setting, assessing your $\dot{V}O2$ max level involves predicting your $\dot{V}O2$ max on the basis of either how well you perform on a specific performance measure (e.g., how fast or how far you walk or run within specific time limits) or how you respond (e.g., your heart rate) to submaximal exercise.

Deciding whether to be tested in a laboratory or a non-laboratory setting and which assessment procedure to use is largely dependent upon the level of testing accuracy that is required, why the testing is being done, what testing resources (personnel and equipment) are available, and what (if any) unique characteristics you might have that would preclude or lend themselves to a specific mode of assessment. You might consider obtaining advice from a health-fitness professional with whom you can discuss your situation and your realistic options for testing.

FAQ #50

Question: In the health and fitness column in my local newspaper, the physician writing the column wrote that in order to get something out of your aerobic conditioning efforts, you have to work out within your "aerobic training zone." To what was she referring?

Answer: Aerobic training zone refers to the training intensity range that will produce improvement in your level of aerobic fitness without overtaxing your cardiorespiratory system. Your aerobic training zone is based on a percentage of your maximal heart rate. As a general rule, your maximal heart rate is measured directly or estimated by subtracting your age from 220. (It is important to note that the method involving subtracting your age from 220 may be associated with considerable error.) Depending upon how physically fit you are, the lower and upper limits of your aerobic training zone are then based on a percentage of the maximal heart rate—approximately 60-90 percent, respectively.

. . . .

FAQ #51

Question: I want to exercise aerobically, but I absolutely do not like running. Is running the best aerobic activity?

Answer: The best aerobic exercise for you (or anyone else for that matter) is one that you enjoy, one that is safe for you, and one that you will engage in on a regular basis. Keep in mind that one person's trash is another person's treasure. In other words, even if you don't want to jog, you can still develop and maintain an adequate level of aerobic fitness. Just pick an aerobic activity that you personally like—exercising on a stair climber, walking on a treadmill, cycling, swimming, etc.—and make it a regular part of your workout regimen. Make sure that your body likes it as much as you do (i.e., the activity doesn't expose your joints and muscles to undue stress).

FAQ #52

Question: What are the "benefits" of stepping backwards on a stair climbing machine? A fitness trainer at my club says such an action will firm and tone my buttocks. Does it?

Answer: Retrograde stair climbing reduces trunk flexion (i.e., forward body lean), thus promoting a more erect and improved body posture during exercise. Many individuals erroneously believe that retrograde stair climbing places a greater emphasis on the gluteal muscles. However, EMG (electromyographic) studies have revealed that retrograde stair climbing places slightly greater (when compared to forward stair climbing) emphasis on the quadriceps (the large group of muscles which make up the front of the thigh) and the hamstrings (muscles on the back of the thigh), while slightly reducing the emphasis placed on the gluteals (large muscles of the buttocks) and gastrocnemius (calves). In our opinion, using a stepping machine in the retrograde position is not justified due to the awkwardness associated with exercising in this manner.

• •

FAQ #53

Question: Does aerobic exercise training significantly strengthen the muscles involved in the activity (e.g., does running significantly strengthen the leg muscles)?

Answer: A regular program of aerobic exercise can produce a number of health benefits, including an increase in aerobic capacity, reduced body weight and fat stores, an improved blood lipid-lipoprotein profile, and lowered arterial blood pressure. For healthy, active adults, however, significant strength gains are not among the benefits of aerobic training. The leg muscles of elite distance runners, for example, have not been found to be significantly stronger than those of healthy, relatively inactive individuals of similar age and gender.

FAQ #54

Question: How fast should my heart beat during an aerobic workout?

Answer: How fast your heart should beat during exercise depends on your age and fitness level (refer to Table 5). According to the American College of Sports Medicine (ACSM), aerobic fitness can best be improved by exercising at an intensity level between 60-90 percent of your maximal heart rate. If you are just starting your workout program, you should exercise at the lower end of the intensity scale (i.e., 60-70 percent). When this level becomes less challenging (usually after three to six months), you should gradually increase the level of exercise intensity until you reach the middle of the range (70-80 percent). As your level of aerobic fitness continues to improve, you may then decide to adjust your exercise intensity rate up towards the higher end of the recommended range (80-90 percent). You should avoid exercising above your target heart rate range, since this could place you at risk for overtraining and/or injury. As a general rule, if you are unable to comfortably carry on a conversation while exercising (a.k.a., the "talk test"), you should reduce your exercise work rate regardless of your heart rate response. Because the "talk test" tends to err on the side of conservatism, and it can be very helpful in ensuring that the intensity of an exercise bout is not excessive for you.

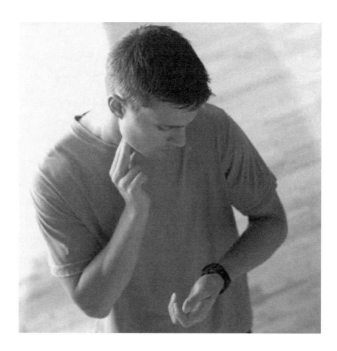

How fast your heart should beat during exercise depends on your age and fitness level.

Table 5. Target Heart Rate Range Chart*

	Relative Fitness Level		
Age	**Low** **(60% - 70%)**	**Middle** **(70% - 80%)**	**High** **(80% - 90%)**
20	20-23	23-26	26-29
25	19-22	22-25	25-28
30	19-22	22-25	25-28
35	18-21	21-24	24-27
40	18-21	21-24	24-27
45	17-20	20-23	23-26
50	17-20	20-23	23-26
55	16-19	19-22	22-25
60	16-19	19-22	22-25
65	16-18	18-21	21-24

* During exercise, count how many times your heart beats in a 10-second interval. Use this chart to see whether your exercise heart rate is in the appropriate range for your age and relative fitness level.

FAQ #55

Question: Does aerobic exercise really help relieve stress?

Answer: Aerobic exercise is one of the most effective "depressurizers" because it helps you dissipate nervous energy and allows your body to metabolize stress-related hormones more rapidly. Any physical activity that involves the major muscles of your body—such as jogging, walking, biking, and swimming—and that is sustained for at least 15 minutes will help to relax your muscles. It will also cause your body to release endorphins, which are naturally produced chemicals that, according to available research, can help relieve stress, impart a sense of well-being, and help you fight off stress-related issues.

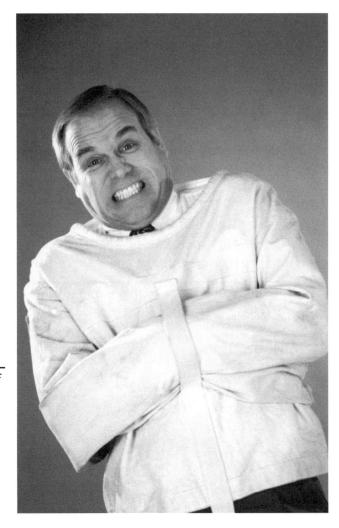

Aerobic exercise is one of the most effective "depressurizers" because it helps you dissipate nervous energy and allows your body to metabolize stress-related hormones more rapidly.

FAQ #56

Question: Can aerobic exercise actually be fun?

Answer: As a point of fact, you should not perceive exercise to be a tortuous expenditure of your time. It should be enjoyable. If you don't find your conditioning regimen to be relatively enjoyable, it is very likely that you will give it up for "greener pastures." Fortunately, almost all individuals can find an exercise activity that both meets their particular needs and is well tolerated—emotionally, as well as physically. Not surprisingly, exercise adherence is always higher (all other factors considered) in those individuals who enjoy what they are doing.

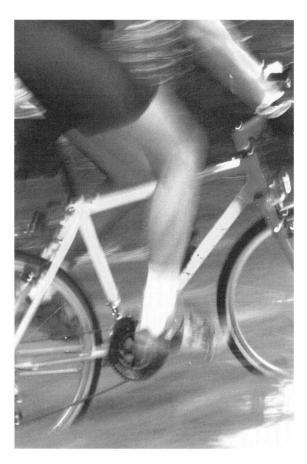

Fortunately, almost all individuals can find an exercise activity that both meets their particular needs and is well tolerated— emotionally, as well as physically.

FAQ #57

Question: What is $\dot{V}O_2$ max and why is it important?

Answer: If you increase the intensity of exercise, a number of things happen in your body. A rise occurs in heart rate, respiration, and oxygen intake, as well as in the activity levels of other parts of your oxygen delivery and utilization (aerobic) systems. A point occurs, however, beyond which oxygen intake cannot increase, even though more work is being performed. At this point, you have reached a level that is commonly referred to as $\dot{V}O_2$ max or maximal oxygen uptake. $\dot{V}O_2$ max is considered to be the best single indicator of aerobic fitness, since it involves the optimal ability of three major systems (pulmonary, cardiovascular, and muscular) of your body to take in, transport, and utilize oxygen. Thus, the higher your $\dot{V}O_2$ max, the greater your level of physical working capacity. Average persons generally have a $\dot{V}O_2$ max of three liters/minute. In contrast, heart patients average 1.5 liters/minute, whereas endurance athletes often range from 5-6 liters/minute.

. . . .

FAQ #58

Question: Is "spinning" a good aerobic conditioning activity?

Answer: "Spinning" is a popular group exercise activity performed on exercise cycles. Typical spinning classes simulate the outdoor cycling experience. Participants maintain very high pedaling rates (at times, as fast as they can pedal) during the workout. The exercise work rate determines the aerobic demand placed on the body (specifically, the cardiovascular and muscular systems). Accordingly, a high heart rate during a spinning workout reflects a relatively substantial level of stress on the body's cardiorespiratory system and, consequently, a significant level of aerobic conditioning. No scientific evidence exists, however, to suggest that spinning is a better aerobic conditioning method than many other popular training modalities (e.g., running, stair climbing, cross-country skiing, etc.).

FAQ #59

Question: On average, who is more aerobically fit—men or women?

Answer: As a general rule, maximal oxygen uptake or $\dot{V}O_2$ max (i.e., an individual's ability to transport and utilize oxygen), considered by most experts to be the best measure of aerobic fitness level, is generally 10-20 percent lower in women. The difference in maximal oxygen uptake between the sexes is smallest when expressed in relative terms (i.e., milliliters of oxygen consumed per kilogram of body weight). This further demonstrates the significance of gender differences in body size. Gender differences in relative maximal oxygen uptake are likely due to differences in cardiac output (i.e., the amount of blood pumped by the heart per minute) and the oxygen-carrying capacity of blood. Women tend to have a decreased ability to deliver blood and oxygen to their exercising muscles because of their smaller lung surfaces, smaller hearts, lower hemoglobin levels in the blood, and reduced muscle mass.

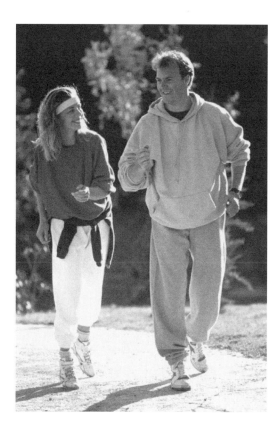

The difference in maximal oxygen uptake between the sexes is smallest when expressed in relative terms.

FAQ #60

Question: Do certain types of strength training significantly enhance a person's level of aerobic fitness?

Answer: A type of strength training known as circuit training has been shown to increase aerobic capacity by an average of approximately five percent—this will vary depending upon the individual's fitness level and how hard the person trains. For example, one study reported that three 20-30 minute circuit training sessions a week for a period of 20 weeks improved aerobic capacity by approximately seven to eight percent—one-third the improvement that might otherwise be expected from a conventional aerobic conditioning program. Some evidence exists, however, that circuit training can be used to effectively maintain improvements in aerobic fitness achieved through traditional forms of aerobic training (i.e., running, cycling, stair climbing, etc.).

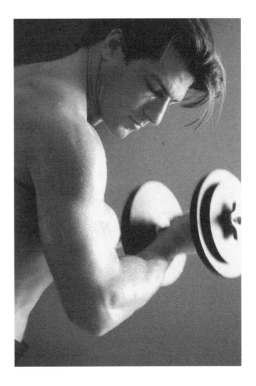

Some evidence exists that shows that circuit training can be used to effectively maintain improvements in aerobic fitness achieved through traditional forms of aerobic training.

FAQ #61

Question: What is cross training and does it offer any significant benefits?

Answer: Cross training is typically defined as an exercise regimen that uses several modes of training to develop a specific component of fitness—in this instance, aerobic fitness. A relatively sound argument can be advanced to support the premise that using two or more types of aerobic exercise in your training regimen is in your best interest. While no evidence exists to support the often stated claim that cross training somehow induces a better aerobic conditioning response, research indicates that using several modes of training can provide an exerciser with positive musculoskeletal and orthopaedic benefits. By combining different exercise modes, you prevent the same bones, muscle groups, and joints from being stressed over and over. As a consequence, cross training tends to reduce the likelihood of your being injured as the result of exercising "too much." In addition, cross training has also been shown to have a positive effect on cardiovascular function (principle of training specificity) and an individual's long-term adherence to a training program.

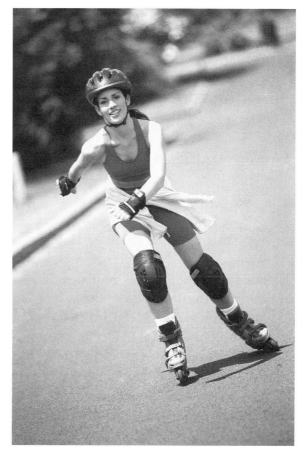

By combining different exercise modes, you prevent the same bones, muscle groups, and joints from being stressed over and over.

FAQ #62

Question: What is a "second wind"?

Answer: No matter how fit you are, the first few minutes into vigorous exercise you'll feel somewhat out of breath, and your muscles may ache. Your body isn't able to transport oxygen to the active muscles quickly enough. As a result, your muscles burn carbohydrates anaerobically causing an increase in lactic acid production. Gradually, your body makes the transition to aerobic metabolism and begins to burn nutrients (carbohydrates and fats) aerobically. This shift over to aerobic metabolism coincides with your getting "back in stride" (a.k.a., the "second wind"). The more you train and the more fit you become, the sooner you will get your "breath" back and reach an aerobic steady state that you can maintain for a relatively extended duration.

● ● ● ● ● ● ● ● ● ● ● ● ● ● ● ● ● ● ● ●

FAQ #63

Question: I sweat profusely (literally dripping wet) during my aerobic workout. Is this an indication that I'm out of shape?

Answer: The reason for profuse sweating is that your body temperature has been significantly elevated by the increase in metabolic heat production during exercise. In response to your elevated body temperature, your brain signals your body to dissipate the excess heat as rapidly as possible. Your sweat glands are then activated, and fluid is transported to your skin so that it can evaporate and cool you off. Rather than indicating a lack of conditioning, sweat dripping off your body may be more indicative of the fact that the humidity of the environment is so high that your sweat can't evaporate. All factors considered, this is not an ideal situation, because it may mean that your body is not being effectively cooled via evaporation. On the other hand, profuse sweating can also be a sign of being relatively fit, since one of the adaptations to consistent exercise training is that individuals will sweat more and sweat sooner so that their bodies don't store extra heat.

FAQ #64

Question: Does in-line skating provide cardiovascular benefits?

Answer: In a word—"yes." Physiologically, your body responds in a manner somewhat similar to running. While in-line skating certainly requires a higher level of motor skills than running, relatively skilled in-line skaters have been found to easily reach and maintain their heart rate in an appropriate training zone while exercising. Accordingly, in-line skating can be a valuable exercise modality for those individuals who are interested in improving their aerobic capacity and/or controlling their body weight.

• •

FAQ #65

Question: Do I need to warm-up and cool-down before a relatively long run?

Answer: Your performance and recovery will be enhanced if you perform a gradual warm-up prior to your exercise regimen and, subsequently, engage in a gradual cool-down program before returning to a resting activity level. Some runners like to finish their training runs with a sprint at the end of the run. This practice can be counter productive. Stopping strenuous exercise abruptly does not offer any positive training benefits and may even be dangerous. If you suddenly stop exercising, blood tends to pool in your legs, placing significant strain on your cardiovascular system as it tries to maintain your level of blood pressure. This response can cause dizziness, fainting, light-headedness, etc. and, in some instances, cardiac failure (i.e., individuals with cardiac abnormalities). By gradually cooling down at the end of your exercise bout (e.g., by engaging in a sprint-jog-walk sequence), you will lessen the strain on your heart and circulatory system while maintaining your blood pressure at a normal level.

FAQ #66

Question: Does bicycling in a very high gear provide a better workout?

Answer: Cycling in a very high gear (which results in a slower pedal cadence and an increase in the force required to turn the pedals) can lead to overuse injuries, such as cyclist's knee. Cyclist's knee is a "catchall" term that refers to pain around or underneath the kneecap. Being forced to push hard on the pedals places considerable stress on the knee joint. On the other hand, pedaling fast in a very low gear may not be preferable either. A fast-paced cadence requires your muscles to contract rapidly. If you haven't been cycling regularly, such a sequence can result in excessive muscle fatigue. Research has shown that the optimal pedal cadence for most recreational cyclists is approximately 60 to 80 revolutions per minute (rpm). Competitive cyclists, on the other hand, typically cycle in the range of 80 to 100 rpm—even faster when they are sprinting. Optimal pedal cadence does vary somewhat from individual to individual, however, depending upon your level of training experience, cycling speed, and the use of accessories (e.g., toe clips). In general, high gears are best used for riding downhill or on level terrain with a good tail wind. Low gears will serve you best if you're climbing a steep hill, carrying gear, or if you have a knee problem that's aggravated by strenuous cycling.

. . . .

FAQ #67

Question: What does the term "aerobic maintenance" mean?

Answer: "Aerobic maintenance" refers to the amount of aerobic exercise you must perform in order to sustain your existing level of aerobic fitness. Most research suggests that you can maintain your level of aerobic fitness by aerobically exercising two or three times weekly at the same level of intensity and duration used to achieve your existing level of fitness.

FAQ #68

Question: What is a rating of perceived exertion and why is it important in aerobic training?

Answer: Being able to listen to your body and to accurately interpret what it's "telling" you regarding the degree of effort you're exerting while exercising aerobically can have positive implications for both your safety and the results you achieve from your training efforts. The most widely accepted measure of sensory input during exercise is the Borg rating of perceived exertion scale (refer to Table 6). Perceived exertion refers to the physical strain individuals believe they are experiencing while exercising. Keep in mind that during exercise, perception of effort is influenced by a variety of cues—some local in nature (e.g., sensations of muscular discomfort or strain) and some central in nature (e.g., heart rate, breathing rate, etc.). Perceived exertion feedback is important because it provides a practical means for individuals to become sensitive to what constitutes an appropriate exercise intensity.

Table 6. The 15-point and 10-point Borg RPE Scales

Category (15-point) RPE Scale		Category/Ratio (10-point) RPE Scale	
6		0	Nothing at all
7	Very, very light	0.5	Very, very weak
8		1	Very weak
9	Very light	2	Weak
10		3	Moderate
11	Fairly light	4	Somewhat strong
12		5	Strong
13	Somewhat hard	6	
14		7	Very strong
15	Hard	8	
16		9	
17	Very hard	10	Very, very strong
18		*	Maximal
19	Very, very hard		
20			

Note: Exercise rated as 11 to 13 (6-20 scale) or 3 to 4 (0-10 scale), between "fairly light" and "somewhat hard" (6-20 scale), or between "moderate" to "somewhat strong" (0-10 scale), is generally appropriate for weight reduction programs, corresponding to about 60 to 70 percent of the maximal heart rate. In contrast, exercise rated 13 to 16 (6-20 scale), between "somewhat hard" and "hard," or 4 to 6 (0-10 scale), between "somewhat strong and very strong," is generally considered more appropriate for cardiorespiratory conditioning, corresponding to 70 to 85 percent of maximal heart rate.

FAQ #69

Question: What is a Metabolic Equivalent (MET)?

Answer: A MET is a unit of measurement that refers to the relative energy demands of an activity in comparison to your energy demands in a resting state. A MET is a multiple of your resting metabolic rate. If you exercise at a 6-MET level, you are exercising at a rate that involves six times the amount of oxygen as your resting state. A MET is estimated to be equal to 3.5 milliliters of oxygen per kilogram of body weight per minute. MET levels can be used to define the energy cost and relative intensity level of any exercise activity (refer to Table 7).

Table 7. Leisure Activities in METs: Sports, Exercise Classes, Games, Dancing

	Mean	Range
Archery	3.9	3-4
Backpacking	—	5-11
Badminton	5.8	4-9+
Basketball		
Gameplay	8.3	7-12+
Non-game	—	3-9
Billiards	2.5	—
Bowling	—	2-4
Calisthenics	—	3-8+
Canoeing, rowing, and kayaking	—	3-8
Climbing hills	7.2	5-10+
Cricket	5.2	4-8
Croquet	3.5	—
Cycling		
Pleasure or to work	—	3-8+
10 mph	7.0	—
Dancing (social, square, tap)	—	3-8
Dancing (aerobic)	—	6-9
Fencing	—	6-10+
Field hockey	8.0	—
Football (touch)	7.9	6-10
Golf		
Power cart	—	2-3
Walking (carrying bag or pulling cart)	5.1	4-7
Handball	—	8-12+
Hiking (cross-country)	—	3-7

Table 7. Leisure Activities in METs: Sports, Exercise Classes, Games, Dancing

	Mean	Range
Horseshoe pitching	—	2-3
Hunting (bow or gun)		
Small game (walking, carrying light load)	—	3-7
Big game (dragging carcass, walking)	—	3-14
Judo	13.5	—
Mountain climbing	—	5-10+
Music playing	—	2-3
Paddleball, racquetball	9	8-12
Rope jumping	11	—
60-80 skips/min	9	—
120-140 skips/min	—	11-12
Running		
12 min per mile	8.7	—
11 min per mile	9.4	—
10 min per mile	10.2	—
9 min per mile	11.2	—
8 min per mile	12.5	—
7 min per mile	14.1	—
6 min per mile	16.3	—
Sailing	—	2.5
Scuba diving	—	5-10
Shuffleboard	—	2-3
Skating, ice and roller	—	5-8
Skiing, snow		
Downhill	—	5-8
Cross-country	—	6-12+
Skiing, water	—	5-7
Sledding, tobogganing	—	4-8
Snowshoeing	9.9	7-14
Squash	—	8-12+
Soccer	—	5-12+
Stair climbing (machine-based)	—	3-17
Swimming	—	4-8+
Table tennis	4.1	3-5
Tennis	6.5	4-9+
Volleyball	—	3-6

Adapted from *ACSM's Guidelines for Exercise Testing and Prescription,* 5th Ed. Baltimore, MD: Williams and Wilkins, 1995.

FAQ #70

Question: How do water-based aerobic activities compare to aerobic workouts performed on land?

Answer: In recent years, an increasing number of individuals have decided to "take to the water" to exercise. While swimming has always enjoyed a certain level of popularity, most of these new water activity advocates have been drawn to a form of exercising that can best be described as "just about every water activity except swimming." Compared to their land-based, aerobic-training counterparts, water exercising offers the following basic benefits to the exerciser:

- *Low impact exercise.* The buoyancy of water facilitates low-impact exercise by effectively reducing an individual's weight (i.e., the proportion of body weight which must be supported) by approximately 90 percent. For example, when a 200-pound man is submerged up to his neck in water, his lower limbs only have to support 20 pounds. As a result, during a workout, that person's joints and ligaments are subjected to substantially less orthopedic stress. Water tends to cushion the impact, not exacerbate the load as a firm surface (e.g., gym floor, sidewalk, roadways, etc.). For example, the orthopedic stress on your skeletal joints while you are running on a non-giving surface has been calculated to be approximately 3-5 times your body weight every time your foot hits. For a 200-pound man who is considering whether or not to exercise in the water or on a solid surface, this translates to a difference between 20 pounds of stress versus at least 600 pounds of orthopedic loading (per step).

- *Minimizes muscular soreness.* Provided that the temperature of the water is relatively comfortable (i.e., between eighty-two and eighty-six degrees Fahrenheit), water appears to have a therapeutic effect. Consequently, while you are exercising in the water, water tends to "massage" your muscles as they are being stretched by the activity. All factors considered, water exercise is an almost painless form of exercise.

- *Applicable to a wide variety of individuals.* Exercising in water can be performed by almost everybody, including many individuals who might otherwise have difficulties with traditional forms of aerobic exercise—in particular, obese individuals, pregnant women, arthritic patients, individuals with preexisting orthopedic conditions (e.g., knees, backs, hips, etc.), and older adults. Fortunately, you do not have to be an Olympic swimmer to exercise in the water. In fact, nonswimmers can safely engage in water exercises—they just have to remain in water no higher than their shoulders. Their heads never have to go under water unless the individuals choose to do so.

- *Relatively inexpensive.* Of course, you need both a bathing suit and access to a swimming pool. Relative to taste, bathing suits are usually affordable. Even if you're not an owner of one of the one and a half million home swimming pools in the United States, you are probably not without an alternative. Access to a pool in which you can exercise is often available at a YMCA, a YWCA, a JCC, a health-fitness facility, a college or university facility, a community-based pool, an apartment-complex pool, etc.

- *Enhances several components of fitness in a single workout.* Depending upon how you design your water exercise program and how physically fit you are, water exercise workouts have the potential to have a positive impact on each of the five basic components of fitness— aerobic fitness, muscular strength, muscular endurance, flexibility, and body composition. In addition, a water exercise workout offers the potential for combined upper and lower extremity training.

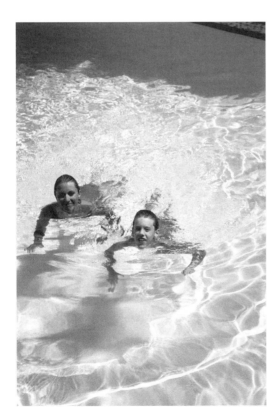

Depending upon how you design your water exercise program and how physically fit you are, water exercise workouts have the potential to have a positive impact on each of the five basic components of fitness.

FAQ #71

Question: Will I get cramps if I eat before I go swimming?

Answer: It is generally safe to go swimming right after eating a light meal. However, it is not a good idea to overeat prior to engaging in any type of strenuous physical activity since blood and oxygen may be diverted from the exercising muscles to the gastrointestinal tract for digestion.

FAQ #72

Question: What causes the pain in my side that occurs suddenly while I am running and how can I prevent it?

Answer: The pain that you've described is referred to as a "side stitch." No clear-cut explanation is universally accepted regarding the painful burning sensation that can occur near the upper portion of the abdominal wall where it meets the rib cage. It has been hypothesized that the side stitch pain is caused by the jarring and pulling on the ligaments that attach the stomach to the diaphragm. Anyone who has experienced a side stitch has probably tried several methods to relieve the pain. While each individual is different, the following methods have been observed to be effective in relieving the pain of a side stitch:

- reducing the exercise intensity level until the pain subsides.
- breathing deeply through pursed lips.
- tightening the abdominal muscles while bending forward.

While you can't totally prevent a side stitch from occurring, you can reduce your likelihood of experiencing one by exercising at an intensity level that matches your fitness level and by gradually increasing how hard you work out as your fitness level improves.

Part II:
Nutrition and
Weight Control

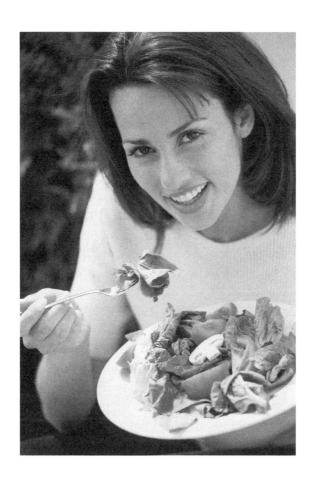

FAQ #73

Question: Obesity is now considered an epidemic in the United States. How did Americans reach this point?

Answer: The answer is complex. Obesity can be caused by several factors, including genetics, hyperphagia (eating too many calories), a high-fat or high-sugar diet, a sluggish metabolic rate, and a sedentary life-style. Hyperplastic obesity is caused by an abnormal increase in the number of fat cells during a person's first year of life and during puberty. An individual of normal weight has about 25 to 30 billion fat cells, while an obese person can have as many as 42 to 106 billion fat cells. With so many reservoirs for fat, it becomes relatively easy for fat to accumulate.

Hyperplastic obesity is rare. Most Americans suffer from hypertrophic obesity in which the number of fat cells is normal, but the size of the cells increases up to 40 percent due to greater fat deposits. Contrary to popular belief, obesity in this country seems to primarily be the result of a sedentary life-style, not overeating. Research shows that obese people don't necessarily eat more than their normal or "healthy" weight counterparts. They simply move less and, therefore, burn fewer calories and store more fat. As they store more fat, the size of their fat cells expands.

Many people who are fat (but not obese) constantly struggle to lose weight as well. Our culture's high premium on thinness has made dieting a way of life for a large segment of the adult population. Because our society imposes such an unrealistic model for the "desirable" physique, many people will try virtually anything to attain a physiologically impossible body weight standard. The demand for quick fixes has encouraged promises of immediate weight loss through nutritionally worthless plans such as fasting, the semi-starvation diet, the all-grapefruit diet, the high-protein, low-carbohydrate diet, the 40-30-30 diet, or even the wood pulp regimen. Not surprisingly, many of these "quick fixes" have been found to cause serious health problems. Admittedly, it is challenging to know who or what to believe.

In reality, all of the tireless efforts to fit into smaller clothing haven't helped the vast horde of dieters shed the pounds and keep them off. As a point of fact, *DIETING ALONE JUST DOESN'T WORK* for most people. Ninety percent of all dieters regain the lost weight within one year and 99 percent within five years. Many are trapped by the "yo-yo" syndrome in which they repeatedly lose and regain the same weight (plus more). The weight loss industry is flourishing simply because no diet gimmick or special food ultimately is successful at long-term weight maintenance.

The only permanent way to effectively lose weight and keep it off is to swear off crash or gimmick diets forever. Instead, all individuals should commit to a lifetime of sound nutritional practices and regular exercise. They should forget promises of instant weight loss and accept the fact that successful weight control requires time, discipline, and perseverance. Although it sounds difficult, the results far outweigh the endless frustration of repeatedly losing and regaining the same pounds.

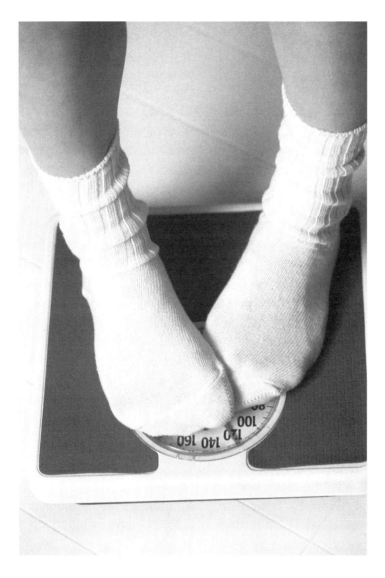

All individuals should commit to a lifetime of sound nutritional practices and regular exercise.

FAQ #74

Question: What is the best method for determining an individual's ideal body weight?

Answer: To determine ideal body weight, individuals should not rely solely on a bathroom scale, height-weight tables, or percent body-fat measurements. Sound nutrition and exercise science principles, along with common sense, mandate that individuals should avoid setting "hard and fast" body-weight goals. Rather, they should strive for achieving a level of body weight that is compatible with a healthy life-style (e.g., sensible eating, regular exercise, etc.). All factors considered, the body weight that results from adopting such a life-style should ultimately be considered as the ideal union between an individual's wellness level, genetic potential, and a state of reality. What represents a safe, realistic, and, perhaps more importantly, attainable body weight for an individual will depend (to a large extent) on the following factors:

- *Medical History*. An individual's current medical history, to include a thoughtful review of personal health-risk factors, should be taken into account when attempting to define ideal body weight. For example, if an individual's blood pressure is elevated, a modest weight reduction (e.g., as little as 10 lbs.) has been shown to be quite beneficial. Extra body mass means that the heart must work harder to pump blood through miles of extra capillaries that feed that extra tissue. Type II diabetes and blood lipid-lipoprotein profiles are further examples of medical conditions that can be positively affected by weight loss.

- *Family History*. Body weight, like most other physical characteristics, is strongly influenced by genetic factors. If an individual's parents and siblings are extremely overweight, it is highly unlikely that such an individual will ever be "model-thin." As unfair as such a judgment might first appear, such a limitation should be kept in mind when establishing ideal body-weight goals.

- *Body Composition*. Leaner bodies are more effective calorie burners. The more muscle or lean body mass individuals have, the more calories they burn. Men naturally have more muscle mass than women, and, as a result, have higher metabolic rates. Furthermore, individuals who exercise on a regular basis tend to have more muscle mass and higher metabolic rates compared with their sedentary counterparts. Accordingly, although individuals who have a relatively high amount of muscle may weigh substantially more than others of similar heights, their body-weight levels may be entirely appropriate given their lean muscle mass.

- *Body-Fat Distribution.* Body fat located in the upper-body region is very risky in terms of health profiles. If individuals possess a high amount of upper-body or abdominal fat, they should consider losing weight (specifically body fat) through a combined program of sensible eating and exercise. One commonly accepted method of determining whether individuals have excessive amounts of upper-body fat is to look at their waist-to-hip ratios. The waist-to-hip ratio (WHR) is a simple, yet accurate, method for determining body-fat distribution patterns. WHR is determined by dividing the waist circumference by the hip circumference. Waist circumference is defined as the smallest circumference between the rib cage and belly button. Hip circumference is defined as the largest circumference of the hip-buttocks region. Men with WHR values exceeding .95 are considered to have an excessive amount of upper-body fat, while those with less than 0.95 are deemed to have an acceptable level of upper-body fat. Women with WHR values above 0.80 are considered to have an unhealthy amount of upper-body fat, while those with scores less than 0.80 are designated as having a reasonable level of accumulated adipose tissue on their upper bodies.

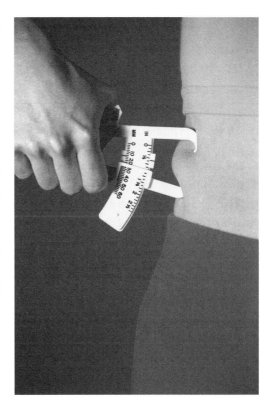

- Functional Ability. If the ability to effectively and efficiently perform activities of daily living and to comfortably engage in a variety of recreational pursuits is impaired, an individual should strive to attain a level of body weight that will support a healthy, functional life-style.

Leaner bodies are more effective calorie burners.

FAQ #75

Question: What is the significance of the waist-to-hip ratio measurement from a health-risk perspective?

Answer: Recent data indicate that the pattern of fat distribution throughout the body is an important predictor of the health risks of obesity. Exercise scientists have classified where the fat is deposited on the body into two basic categories: male-pattern (or apples) and female-pattern (or pears). Despite their names, each type of fat pattern can occur in both sexes, although men tend to be apples and women tend to be pears. Apples characteristically deposit high amounts of fat in the abdominal and trunk regions, while pears deposit high amounts of fat in the hip, buttocks, and thigh regions.

The waist-to-hip ratio (WHR) is a simple, yet accurate, method for determining your body fat pattern. WHR is determined by dividing the waist circumference by the hip circumference. Waist circumference is defined as the smallest circumference between the rib cage and belly-button. Hip circumference is defined as the largest circumference of the hip-buttocks region.

Men with WHR values exceeding 0.95 are considered apples; those with less than 0.95 are deemed pears. Women with WHR values above 0.80 are considered apples, those with scores less than 0.80 are designated as pears. Research has shown that apples are at a greater risk for developing a number of health-related problems, the most prominent being hypertension (i.e., high blood pressure), type II diabetes (i.e., non-insulin dependent diabetes), and hyperlipidemia (i.e., elevated levels of fat in the blood).

Scientists believe that two characteristics of abdominal fat cells are probably responsible for the greater health risk associated with being an apple. Abdominal fat cells tend to be larger than those located in other regions of the body. Relatively large fat cells are associated with insulin resistance (i.e., reduced tissue responsiveness to insulin), which means body cells will take up less glucose (sugar) from the blood, causing the blood sugar level to rise. In response to the elevated blood sugar level, the pancreas secretes more and more insulin (hyperinsulinemia). Full-blown diabetes (type II) can develop if blood sugar rises enough.

Hyperinsulinemia, by promoting sodium reabsorption by the kidneys and stimulating the sympathetic nervous system, can predispose an apple to hypertension. Also, the rates of enzyme-initiated chemical reactions are higher for abdominal fat cells, thus making them more metabolically active than fat cells located in other regions of the body. The more metabolically active abdominal fat cells can be easily released into the blood stream resulting in hyperlipidemia.

All the news is not bad for apples, however. Research has shown that weight reduction tends to be easier for them, as they benefit from the high turnover rate of abdominal fat. For pears, however, weight loss is more difficult because fat cells in the hip, buttock, and thigh regions do not easily relinquish their fat. This tendency for pears to stubbornly hold onto their fat helps to ensure that nursing mothers maintain sufficient energy reserves. While it is true that apples are at a greater health risk and pears are at a disadvantage with regard to weight reduction, exercise training and a prudent diet (regardless of your body shape) can help to counteract many of the negative health consequences of obesity and result in a weight loss that can be maintained.

* *

FAQ #76

Question: What causes cellulite, and what, if anything, can be done to eliminate it? Do any of the creams, herbs, wraps, antitoxins, or special exercises actually work?

Answer: When the fibrous strands within ordinary fat tissue become stretched, they produce a dimpling effect on the overlying skin. The dimpled appearance, often seen on the hips, thighs, and buttocks, is commonly referred to as cellulite by the plethora of manufacturers, marketers, and sellers of the various gimmicks and gadgets that purportedly work to remove it. However, nothing unique exists about that kind of fat on the body. Short of liposuction, no special or "secret" methods—including creams, foods, diets, drugs, machines, or exercises—will selectively eliminate the so-called cellulite.

FAQ #77

Question: Please settle an argument. Is beer a good post-workout drink?

Answer: It may taste good when you're thirsty, but beer is not an effective way to rehydrate after exercising. Alcohol has a diuretic effect. As a result, instead of replenishing fluids, beer promotes additional water loss via urination. In reality, the diuretic effect of beer can lead to hypohydration or, in severe cases, dehydration. Some individuals believe that beer gives them a carbohydrate boost plus extra potassium. An urgent need for these nutrients immediately following a workout doesn't exist, however. Even if an individual needed these particular nutrients, beer is a relatively poor source. For example, compared to orange juice, beer has only 13 grams and 89 milligrams of carbohydrates and potassium, respectively, versus 39 grams of carbohydrates and 700 milligrams of potassium in orange juice.

•••••••••••••••••••••

FAQ #78

Question: Is it true that aerobic exercise burns fat faster than other types of exercise?

Answer: Aerobic exercise is the only way for your body to burn fat directly. Anaerobic exercise uses only carbohydrates, while aerobic exercise uses carbohydrates and fats. At a point after approximately 20 minutes of aerobic exercise, your body shifts from using mainly carbohydrates as fuel to using more fats. You need to keep in mind, however, that when you eat, you replenish both carbohydrates and fats. As soon as you reach a point of having consumed an excess of calories, your body begins to store those calories as fat. If you eat after an activity that utilizes more fats than carbohydrates, you fill up your carbohydrate stores faster, thereby creating a situation where the excess calories are converted to fat anyway. Thus, you haven't altered your body's overall caloric balance. You lose weight when you expend more calories than you consume, not because you burn fat when you work out.

FAQ #79

Question: Will wearing rubberized shirts and pants or extra layers of clothing to increase sweating help me lose extra pounds of body fat during my aerobic workouts?

Answer: Extra layers of clothing and rubberized sweatsuits can elevate body temperature (because such clothing inhibits evaporative heat loss) and cause increased sweating. No matter how hot you become, however, sweating does not significantly increase the number of calories burned, which is how fat weight is lost. Any weight loss you might experience following a workout in a rubberized suit is the result of lost water, not lost body fat. As soon as you replace the water through drinking and/or eating, the lost pounds quickly return.

· · · · · · · · · · · · · · · · · · · ·

FAQ #80

Question: Does an aerobic workout cause an individual's resting metabolic rate to stay elevated for a long time after a workout (the so-called "after burn" effect)?

Answer: In general, the available scientific data indicate that the amount of energy expended after an aerobic workout tends to be very small. The number of calories burned during the recovery is dependent upon the intensity and the duration of the workout. Following exercise of unusual intensity and duration, your metabolic rate may remain elevated for as long as 24 hours—but at levels that are just barely above resting baseline levels. In general, approximately 15 extra calories are burned during recovery for every 100 calories expended during an exercise bout.

FAQ #81

Question: Does aerobic exercise have a positive effect on the reduction in resting metabolism associated with dieting?

Answer: Most available research suggests that moderate-intensity aerobic exercise training does little to diminish the usual 10-20 percent diet-induced reduction in resting metabolic rate (RMR). In fact, some studies indicate that combining aerobic exercise with a very low-calorie diet (less than 1000 calories per day) stimulates the body to conserve energy, thereby signaling the body to initiate the process of decreasing the RMR.

· ·

FAQ #82

Question: I'm interested in losing weight. What type of exercise is best?

Answer: It takes two different types of exercise to help you most effectively lose weight and keep it off: one to burn a high number of calories (aerobic-type exercise), the other to build and preserve muscle tissue (strength-training exercise). Muscle tissue enables you to lose weight and keep it off because it helps you maintain your resting metabolic rate, thereby allowing you to burn a greater number of calories when you're at rest. An analysis of the available data indicates that, in general, the combination of a conventional aerobic exercise program with a severely calorie-restricted diet does little (if anything) to help preserve lean body mass during weight reduction.

It is important to keep in mind that the less lean body mass you have, the lower your resting metabolic rate will be. As a result, it is more likely that you will regain some or all of the weight loss you may have achieved. On the other hand, if you engage in exercise designed to improve your muscular fitness level at the same time you are losing weight, you will enhance the likelihood that you will be able to maintain your level of lean body mass. As a consequence, the optimal exercise prescription for sound weight management is one that combines aerobic conditioning and strength training.

FAQ #83

Question: Will I lose body fat more efficiently by performing my aerobic workouts at a low, rather than a high, intensity?

Answer: Many aerobic exercise programs and videos feature low-intensity workouts which purport to maximize fat burning. The argument behind such an alleged theory is that low-intensity aerobic training will allow your body to use more fat as an energy source, thereby accelerating the loss of body fat. While it is true that a higher proportion of calories burned during low-intensity exercise come from fat (about 60 percent as opposed to approximately 35 percent from high-intensity programs), high-intensity exercise still burns more calories from fat in the final analysis. For example, if you perform thirty minutes of low-intensity aerobic exercise (i.e., at a level of 50 percent of maximal exercise capacity), you'll burn approximately 200 calories—about 120 of those come from fat (i.e., 60 percent). However, exercising for the same amount of time at a high intensity (i.e., 85 percent of your maximal exercise capacity) will burn approximately 400 calories. Using a 35 percent fat utilization yardstick, 140 of the calories you've burned will have come from stored fat.

Although the more vigorous exercise burns both more total and more fat calories, the less intense form of exercise has its benefits as well. For example, because many overweight people tend to find that lower-intensity exercise is more comfortable, they may, therefore, be willing to engage in such workouts. The point to remember is that low-intensity workouts do, in fact, promote weight and fat loss. You just have to do them for a longer period of time.

Low-intensity aerobic exercise, however, is not a better or more effective way to lose weight than more intense physical activity—the idea of a "fat-burning zone" is simply a myth. Keep in mind that you lose weight and body fat when you expend more calories than you consume, not because you burn fat (or anything else) when you exercise.

FAQ #84

Question: I've heard from several marathon runners that I should "carbohydrate load" to improve my performance. What is carbohydrate loading and does it work?

Answer: Some marathoners practice "carbohydrate loading" in their diets to improve performance. They believe that stored carbohydrate (glycogen) is important to sustained, higher intensity performance. Available research generally supports the contention that increased carbohydrate intake (sugars and starches) results in improved athletic performance—particularly in long-duration endurance activities such as a marathon. The individual with adequate muscle glycogen stores will be able to perform for a longer period of time at a higher intensity or pace. The body relies on fat as the major fuel source during mild exercise. But, as the intensity of the exercise bout (i.e., running faster) is increased, the body relies increasingly on carbohydrates—largely because carbohydrates provide the greatest energy yield. During a prolonged bout of exercise, the body may utilize all of its limited carbohydrate reserves. While you may be able to continue exercising, you will have to decrease your running speed. Trying to run at faster speeds while burning fat will result in fatigue and muscular exhaustion.

   To reach the highest pre-competition level of muscle glycogen, most experts recommend that you first deplete your glycogen stores through an exhaustive bout of prolonged exercise. You should do this approximately one week prior to the competition. For the next four days, you should attempt to maintain these low glycogen storage levels by continued training and a diet predominantly composed of fat and protein. The three days before the competition should be reserved for a carbohydrate-rich diet, combined with mild or low-intensity workouts. This type of regimen produces an "overshoot phenomenon," resulting in the greatest possible glycogen storage in the muscles. It is best to experiment with carbohydrate loading before trying it prior to a competition because it is not without side effects. Undesirable side effects associated with carbohydrate loading include marked physical and mental fatigue, elevation of fat metabolic by-products in the blood, low blood sugar levels, EKG abnormalities, depression, irritability, and bloating.

FAQ #85

Question: Why does aerobic exercise have minimal effect in accelerating weight loss when combined with a low-calorie diet?

Answer: Several possible reasons exist for why aerobic exercise does little to accelerate weight loss when combined with a low-calorie diet. Among the more commonly cited reasons are the following:

• Many overweight/overfat individuals are unable to perform high amounts of exercise without subjecting their bodies to an undue level of orthopedic stress—thereby incurring an injury. High amounts of exercise are needed to promote weight loss, but the risk of orthopedic injury limits the amount of exercise that can be safely performed by many overweight/overfat individuals.

• The "net caloric expenditure" of moderate aerobic workouts is relatively small. The net calorie cost of exercise is equal to the number of calories expended during an exercise bout that are used beyond the number of calories expended by an individual's resting metabolism (RMR) and other activities that the individual might have engaged in had he/she otherwise not been exercising (refer to Table 8).

• Some individuals who exercise tend to reward themselves by resting and relaxing more after their workouts are over. As a result, the net change in their total 24-hour caloric expenditure levels may be virtually unchanged.

Table 8. The Net Caloric Expenditure of a 4-Mile Walk in 1 Hour by a 150 lb. Person

Variable	Calories Expended
Gross Caloric Expenditure for a 4-Mile Walk	320 Calories
Resting Metabolic Rate for 1 Hour	-70 Calories
Caloric Expenditure for Mild Physical Activity the Person Might Have Engaged in Had He/She Not Been Formally Walking	-70 Calories
Net Caloric Expenditure of a 4-Mile Walk*	180 Calories

*Note: One pound equals 3,500 calories.

FAQ #86

Question: Does aerobic exercise counter the decrease in lean muscle mass associated with dieting?

Answer: In general, the combination of a moderate-intensity aerobic exercise program with a low-calorie diet does little to protect lean muscle mass during weight loss. During weight loss, the percentage of weight lost as lean muscle mass increases in direct proportion to the magnitude of the calorie deficit encountered by the body. As a result of rigorous fasting, the total body weight that is lost is approximately 50 percent fat and 50 percent lean muscle mass. During a very low-calorie diet (with adequate protein intake), the proportions improve to 75 percent fat and 25 percent lean muscle mass. During a low-calorie diet (approximately 1200-1500 calories per day), the proportions improve even more to 90 percent fat and only 10 percent lean muscle mass. Moderate-intensity aerobic exercise, on the other hand, has been found to have a very limited effect on these body composition proportions. Resistance training during weight loss, however, has been shown to provide a sufficient stimulus to offer protection against the loss of the lean muscle mass during sensible dieting.

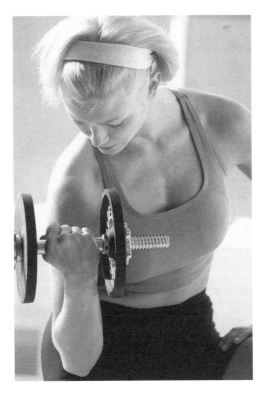

During weight loss, the percentage of weight lost as lean muscle mass increases in direct proportion to the magnitude of the calorie deficit encountered by the body.

FAQ #87

Question: If aerobic exercise doesn't help me to lose weight much faster, then why should I spend the extra time and effort running, stair climbing, cycling, etc.?

Answer: Despite its limitations with regard to promoting weight loss, exercising aerobically provides several important health benefits. Among the major health benefits of aerobic exercise for overweight/overfat individuals are the following:

- Improved aerobic capacity. All other factors being equal, an individual with a high aerobic capacity will have a high physical working capacity.

- Reduced risk of developing obesity-related diseases such as diabetes, coronary heart disease, and hypertension.

- Improved blood lipid-lipoprotein profile, specifically decreased triglycerides, and increased high density lipoprotein cholesterol (HDL-C)—the "good" form.

- Improved psychological status, particularly enhanced self-esteem, general well-being, and decreased anxiety and depression.

- Increased fat loss to weight loss ratio (i.e., more of the weight lost is fat).

- Enhanced long-term weight management. Regular exercise is the most powerful predictor of long-term weight loss success. It helps to ensure that individuals not only lose weight, but also keep it off.

FAQ #88

Question: Is there a quick and easy "weigh" to lose weight?

Answer: In a word, no. Almost all diets share at least one common trait—eventually, they don't work. To lose weight and keep it off (the really difficult part of controlling your weight), you must be willing to incorporate permanent changes in both your eating habits and your physical activity level. In addition to a formal exercise program, physical activity must be increased in your daily living.

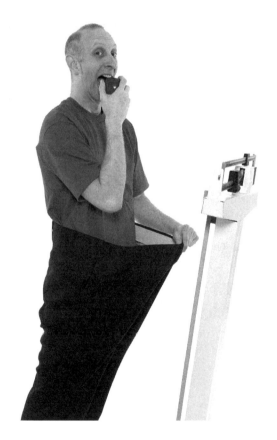

Almost all diets share at least one common trait—eventually, they don't work.

FAQ #89

Question: Could you please explain what is the "set point theory" as it relates to weight control?

Answer: Many nutritional and weight control experts hypothesize that an individual's overall level of body weight and level of relative body fatness can be affected by a number of conditions. One particular factor that is believed to play an important role in this regard is commonly referred to as an individual's "set point." Proponents of the set point theory claim that the body has an internal control mechanism that is located deep within the hypothalamus of the brain that drives the body to maintain a particular level of body fat. When the amount of stored body fat falls outside the set point range (either increases or decreases), the brain makes the necessary adjustments in both an individual's appetite and metabolic rate until the amount of stored body fat, once again, falls within the set point range. Accordingly, this physiological feedback mechanism determines the amount of fat an individual's body sustains. A higher set point results in more fat stored, while a lower set point causes less fat to be stored.

All factors considered, it is believed that dieting tends to increase an individual's set point range, because it usually results in the loss of lean body mass (LBM) that causes a concomitant decrease in metabolic rate. Over time, this process often leads to the "yo-yo" syndrome in which perpetual dieters continue to eat too few calories and, in the absence of resistance exercise, to significantly reduce their levels of LBM. As a result of the effect that their diminished level of LBM has on their metabolic rate, they also continue to store more body fat. Faced with a succession of higher set points, these individuals tend to encounter more difficulty losing weight. With each successive diet, they tend to repeatedly lose and regain the same pounds.

An important factor to keep in mind is that according to proponents of the set point theory, the most effective way to lower an individual's set point—and, therefore, that person's level of stored fat—is through exercise. Research has shown that the best program of exercise for sound weight control is one that combines both aerobic exercise and resistance training.

FAQ #90

Question: Does aerobic exercise suppress a person's appetite? Some experts say it does, others say it doesn't. Who is right?

Answer: The vast majority of studies have demonstrated that caloric intake is usually unchanged or slightly increased in response to long-term aerobic exercise training. Energy intake is, however, usually increased below the level of the increase in energy expenditure. This situation results in a negative energy balance (i.e., energy expenditure > energy intake) and, concomitantly, a loss of body weight and body fat. Some evidence exists, however, that if you vigorously exercise before you eat, you will actually eat less because of an increase in your body temperature and an alteration in your hormone levels. Other studies suggest that moderate exercise actually decreases the appetite among previously sedentary adults. Keep in mind that the centers for the thermoregulatory system, appetite, and sleep lie right next to each other in the brain stem. When you affect one, you will likely affect the others.

• •

FAQ #91

Question: Should I eat breakfast before going for my morning run?

Answer: Ideally, you want to achieve a situation where you avoid feeling hungry during your workout without feeling too full. Eating a light breakfast consisting of carbohydrate-rich foods or beverages (e.g., toast, fruit, or juices) an hour before your workout should provide a sufficient number of calories to keep you energized during your run. Consuming a large breakfast (particularly one that is high in fat and/or protein) prior to exercise is not recommended because when you start exercising, the digestion process slows down, which could lead to gastrointestinal distress and stomach discomfort.

FAQ #92

Question: Should aerobically active individuals take supplemental forms of antioxidants?

Answer: All factors considered, the jury is still out on whether an individual should take antioxidant supplements. On one hand, the renowned founder and president of the Cooper Institute for Aerobics Research (based in Dallas, Texas), Kenneth Cooper, M.D., claims that individuals who exercise regularly need antioxidant supplements more than ever. Other scientists—in an attempt to examine Cooper's largely anecdotal-documented claims—have conducted scientifically controlled studies, which have produced results that actually refute Cooper's recommendations.

Both sides of the argument tend to agree that relatively large amounts of exercise (e.g., more than five hours per week) will increase the body's production of free radicals (minute reactive chemicals that are produced in response to a cell's natural process of using oxygen for metabolism). In the long run, an excessive level of free radicals, if left unchecked, can cause irreparable harm to the body, including an increased risk of heart disease and some types of cancer. By neutralizing free radicals, antioxidants may protect the body's cells from damage. Many noted medical and nutritional experts contend that the best defense against free radical damage is to consume antioxidants—particularly beta carotene, vitamin C, and vitamin E—which are chemical compounds either produced by the body or obtained from foods.

Based upon unpublished data gathered at the Cooper Institute, Cooper has been at the forefront of a relatively small group of medical and nutritional experts who advocate taking megadoses of antioxidant supplements on a daily basis. Cooper's detractors (in the matter) point to the results of a recently published six-year study conducted by Finnish physicians to support their contention that antioxidant supplementation may not be all that it's purported to be. Surprisingly, this investigation found that supplements of vitamin E and beta carotene may actually increase, rather than decrease, a smoker's risk of cancer, stroke, and heart disease.

In reality, until more controlled research is conducted on the issue, you should strongly consider taking a middle road between the two extreme positions on antioxidant supplementation. In other words, you should eat as many foods rich in antioxidants as you feel is feasible. Subsequently, if you feel that your diet is not providing you with enough antioxidants, then take an antioxidant supplement—but only in moderation.

Avoid the "more-must-be-better" megadose approach. Taking megadoses of antioxidants (or any other vitamins) is not advocated by most health and nutrition experts, because some vitamins, when taken in megadoses, can be toxic or cause serious adverse side effects, and the long-term effects are largely unknown.

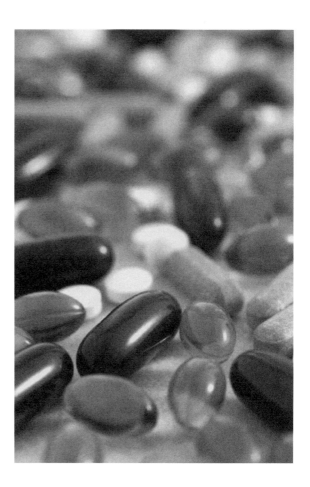

Taking megadoses of antioxidants (or any other type of vitamin) is not advocated by most health and nutrition experts.

FAQ #93

Question: Several people at the gym that I go to say that creatine supplements will increase the size and strength of my muscles. Is this true?

Answer: Creatine is certainly one of the hot supplements among fitness enthusiasts. A growing body of evidence exists to suggest that taking creatine supplements may improve a person's ability to perform short-term, intense exercise. All skeletal muscle tissue contains creatine, and dietary creatine is found in meat and fish. During exercise, a portion of the muscle's creatine is depleted. Creatine phosphate plays an important role in resynthesizing ATP during short bursts of high-intensity exercise. Creatine supplements have been shown to increase the total creatine content (creatine and creatine phosphate) of muscle on an average of 20-30 percent. Several studies suggest that ingestion of 20-25 grams of creatine monohydrate per day for 5-6 days improves muscular performance during activities that require high levels of strength and power (e.g., weight lifting, sprinting). Sufficient evidence exists to state that, under certain conditions, creatine supplementation can enhance performance in activities that require short periods of high-intensity power and strength. If individuals can train at higher intensity levels, it follows that they may be able to add strength and power at accelerated rates over a period of time. Creatine can also lead to weight gain, but the mechanism responsible for the added weight has not been adequately investigated. Before you run out and start taking creatine supplements, consider the following precautions:

- The long-term effects of taking creatine have not been studied. The majority of studies have examined the effect of the short-term (30 days or less) use of creatine.

- All the studies conducted have involved adults only. Creatine's effects on children are unknown.

- Consuming large quantities of creatine (greater than 30 grams per month) may encourage fat to accumulate in the liver.

- Stomach cramping and diarrhea have been cited as adverse side effects of creatine supplementation.

FAQ #94

Question: I run 2-3 miles on 3-4 days per week; do I need to take extra vitamins?

Answer: The vitamin needs of an active person are generally no greater than those of a sedentary one. Vitamins do not contribute significantly to your body's structure and do not provide you with a direct source of body energy, so physically active people receive no benefit from taking excessive amounts of vitamin supplements. If you eat a variety of healthful foods (breads, cereals, grains, fruits, vegetables, lean meats, etc.), your intake of vitamins will be adequate.

. . . .

FAQ #95

Question: What exactly is chromium, and does it really help people gain muscle and lose fat?

Answer: Chromium is an essential trace mineral in the body that aids insulin in the transfer of glucose from the bloodstream into the cells. It also plays a role in fat metabolism. Chromium picolinate, a supplemental form of chromium, has gained widespread popularity recently as a potent stimulus for simultaneous muscular development and fat loss. Despite claims to the contrary, little reliable evidence exists to suggest that chromium deficiency is a widespread problem. This is not surprising since chromium is found in water, beverages, and practically everything we eat. The few research studies that have been conducted using sound methodologies have not found a beneficial effect of chromium supplementation on levels of either lean muscle mass or body fat. In November 1996, the Federal Trade Commission (FTC) forced three of the leading marketers of chromium picolinate to stop making undocumented claims, including the assertion that the pills promote weight loss, burn fat, build muscle, lower cholesterol, regulate blood sugar, and treat or prevent diabetes. The FTC concluded that these health claims had not been substantiated by scientific studies, and that no reliable evidence existed for the claim that most Americans don't consume enough chromium in their diets.

FAQ #96

Question: Do aerobically active individuals need to take mineral supplements?

Answer: About four percent of your body's weight is composed of a group of 22 metallic elements collectively called minerals. Although not all minerals are essential for life, most are present in living cells. The minerals of greatest importance to humans are those present in hormones, enzymes, and vitamins. Minerals are found in muscles, connective tissues, and all body fluids.

Minerals serve several roles in your body. Their single most critical role is their involvement in cellular metabolism. As an integral part of the enzymes that regulate chemical reactions within cells, selected minerals participate in the catabolic and anabolic cellular processes that are crucial to normal physiological functioning. Minerals also constitute a critical part of your body's hormones. Inadequate levels of specific minerals in your hormones could have dire consequences for you (e.g., the hormone that facilitates glucose uptake by the cells requires zinc).

For a variety of reasons, many individuals do not eat a balanced diet. In those instances, taking a basic "one-a-day" vitamin/mineral tablet may be appropriate. For most individuals, however, little need exists for supplementing their diet with minerals because most minerals are readily found in water and a well-balanced diet. By the same token, no evidence exists that for individuals who ingest the recommended daily allowance of minerals, that excess mineral supplementation benefits their exercise performance or enhances their recovery from exercise.

FAQ #97

Question: Are some carbohydrates better sources of energy than others?

Answer: In reality, with regard to serving as a source of energy, all carbohydrates are not all the same. Some release energy quickly. Others do it over a longer period of time. To determine which foods provide quick energy versus those that will keep energy levels high until an individual's next meal, it helps to understand the Glycemic Index (GI) which assigns a value to each food indicating how fast energy will be released.

White bread—the standard by which foods are judged—is assigned a GI of 100. Foods with a relatively low GI rating (i.e., 75 or less) release energy gradually. On the other hand, foods with a rating of greater than 75 provide a comparatively faster energy boost that tends to fade fairly quickly. (Note: the higher the GI rating, the faster the energy is released.) A list of the GI ratings of an average serving size for some commonly consumed foods is provided in Table 9. When selecting the food choice for a "carbo load," individuals should decide when they want the energy to kick in—sooner or later?

Table 9. Glycemic Index for Various Foods

Puffed rice cereal	132	All-bran cereal	74
Honey	126	Kidney beans	71
Cornflakes	121	Orange juice	71
White bread	100	Ice cream	69
Corn chips	99	Rye or wheat bread	68
Mashed potatoes	98	Frozen green peas	65
Raisins	93	Macaroni	64
Carrots	92	Spaghetti	61
Oatmeal	90	Yogurt	52
Banana	84	Skim milk	46
Most types of cookies	80	Most fruits	42
Sweet corn	80	Fructose	30
Potato chips	77	Peanuts	15

FAQ #98

Question: I've had a few clients lose significant amounts of weight by following the zone diet. Does this diet actually work?

Answer: Proponents of the zone diet advocate a dietary approach that is relatively balanced in which 40 percent of calories should come from carbohydrates, 30 percent from fat, and 30 percent from protein. The 40-30-30 theory centers on insulin, a hormone that helps blood glucose get into muscle cells, where it is used as energy. Carbohydrates stimulate the release of insulin which, in turn, encourages the entrance of glucose into cells. Since insulin inhibits the use of fat, a high level of insulin in the bloodstream prevents the breakdown of fat for energy. What the proponents of the zone diet fail to fully understand are the synergistic components of the process of energy balance.

When calories consumed are equal to the amount of energy required, no need exists for fat stores to be burned. In other words, supply and demand dictate whether carbohydrate is used immediately as an energy source or stored for later use as glycogen or fat. If the amount of calories consumed as carbohydrates, fat, or protein exceed the amount of energy expended, the excess energy will be stored as fat. Since eating and exercising are not done simultaneously, sustained exercise always relies on the limited supply of stored energy from glycogen, along with the more abundant supply of body fat. During aerobic exercise that lasts for a relatively long period of time, the human body adapts for increased fat utilization, thereby enabling individuals to exercise longer without experiencing undue fatigue or exhaustion.

Stored fat, however, can only provide approximately 50 percent of the required energy with carbohydrate providing the rest. As a result, a diet that supplies only 40 percent of its calories from carbohydrate may be unsatisfactory for a physically active person because it may limit glycogen storage and, consequently, endurance. The 40-30-30 nutrient mix may require that a portion of protein be used as energy rather than for its chief function of helping to build and maintain body tissue. This use of protein as an energy source also increases the risk of dehydration since the metabolic waste products from protein breakdown are eliminated via the urine. In reality, people tend to lose weight on the 40-30-30 diet simply because they are low in calories (e.g., a typical male on the zone diet would consume approximately 1700 calories per day and female about 1300 calories per day)—not because they offer any "magical features."

FAQ #99

Question: Are there any risks associated with excess protein consumption?

Answer: The human body is unable to store extra protein. Protein consumed in excess of the body's needs is not used to build muscle; rather, it is used for non-protein bodily functions. If individuals consume protein in excess of their caloric and protein needs, the extra protein will not be stored as protein. Unfortunately such extra protein is converted to and stored as fat. As a result, if individuals consume large amounts of extra protein, in addition to their regular dietary intake, any weight gain would very likely be in the form of fat.

Another important point to keep in mind is that the potential for harm exists if protein is consumed in excess. Such harm is most likely to occur in the individual who consumes protein or amino acid supplements. For example, excess protein may lead to dehydration, because protein metabolism requires extra water for utilization and excretion (i.e., elimination) of its by-products. Since exercising individuals are already at an increased risk for dehydration, the additional strain of protein waste excretion may further promote dehydration. Excess protein has also been shown to lead to an increase in the loss of urinary calcium. A chronic calcium loss, due to excess protein intake, is of particular concern because it may increase the risk of osteoporosis, especially in women.

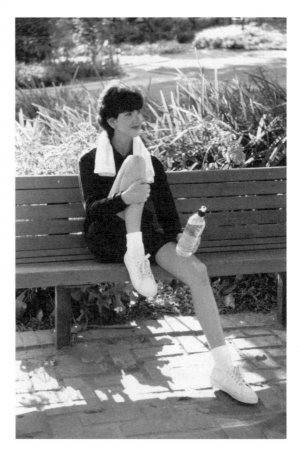

Excess protein may lead to dehydration.

FAQ #100

Question: How much protein do athletes really require?

Answer: At least two issues need to be addressed when discussing the protein needs of an athlete: protein as a source of fuel and protein for building muscle mass. Early research conducted on these issues surmised that because muscles include considerable protein that it must be their preferred fuel. Furthermore, it was inferred that increases in muscle mass must come from extra dietary protein. It is now known, however, that carbohydrates, in the form of muscle glycogen, are the primary fuel for muscles. Research also confirms that sound resistance training builds and strengthens muscles, not extra dietary protein.

Even though most exercise scientists agree with current research, they believe that protein plays an important secondary role during exercise that may increase an athlete's need for protein above the recommended daily allowance (RDA). The American Dietetic Association (ADA) recommends increased protein intake only for individuals involved in intense aerobic training (greater than 70 percent $\dot{V}O2$ max). Even though the ADA developed such a recommendation, it recognizes that average Americans, including most athletes, consume protein above this recommendation.

The ADA does not support the notion that the protein needs of a competitive weight-lifter are greater than the average individual. The official ADA position is that a well-balanced diet will provide the dietary protein a weight lifter needs. Accordingly, an individual who would like to add muscle should focus on combining a sound resistance-training program with a well-balanced, calorically dense diet.

Most exercise scientists and dietitians agree that exercise does not increase the body's need for protein significantly. A few, however, believe that physically active individuals have an increased need for protein. Peter Lemon, Ph.D., professor of applied physiology at Kent State University, Kent, Ohio, is a renowned advocate of the theory of increased protein needs for athletes. He recommends that athletes consume between one to one-and-a-half times more protein than the established RDA. On the other hand, since average Americans, including most athletes, already consume one-and-a-half to two times the RDA, it would appear that athletes do not need to increase their protein intake.

FAQ #101

Question: What is androstenedione and is it a safe alternative to anabolic steroids?

Answer: Androstenedione is a steroid that can be converted to testosterone. It is produced naturally by the body. It is also marketed and sold
as a natural supplement under various trade names, despite the fact that no
medical reason exists for taking it. Marketers and manufacturers of androstenedione claim that a 100-milligram dose of androstenedione can increase
plasma concentrations of testosterone by a factor of four within 90 minutes.
Additional claims concerning this supplement are that "andro" (as it is popu-
larly referred to among users) increases muscle size, strength, energy, im-
mune function, libido (sex drive), and general well-being.

Many experts believe that, as with other steroids, androstenedione
improves the body's ability to rapidly recover from strenuous physical activity, thereby allowing its users to train more frequently at higher levels of
intensity. The result of such training efforts presumably would be an increase in muscle size and strength. Dr. Charles Yesalis, a leading expert on
the topic of anabolic steroids, contends that androstenedione should be
placed on the list of substances covered by the Anabolic Steroid Control Act
of 1990 and its use controlled until the long-term health consequences
associated with it are determined. It should also be kept in mind that
despite the fact that androstenedione is sold legally over-the-counter, it is
banned by the National Collegiate Athletic Association, the International
Olympic Committee, and the National Football League. Nonetheless, androstenedione received considerable attention in 1998 because of its much-
publicized use by Mark McGuire in his home run, record-breaking season.